Dressing Modern
Like Our Mothers

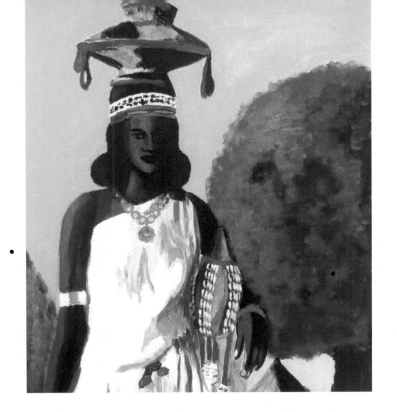

Dressing Modern Like Our Mothers

Dress, Identity, and Cultural Praxis in Oromia

Peri M. Klemm

THE RED SEA PRESS

TRENTON | LONDON | NEW DELHI | CAPE TOWN | NAIROBI | ADDIS ABABA | ASMARA | IBADAN

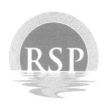

THE RED SEA PRESS
541 West Ingham Avenue | Suite B
Trenton, New Jersey 08638

Book design: Dawid Kahts
Cover design: Asharful Haq
Book cover artwork: Yadesa Bojia

Library of Congress Cataloging-in-Publication Data may be obtained from the Library of Congress.

ISBNs: 978-1-56902-780-6 (HB)
        978-1-56902-781-3 (PB)

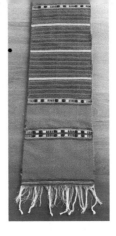

Table of Contents

Figures

Abbreviations

AIDS	Acquired Immune Deficiency Syndrome
EPLF	Eritrean People's Liberation Front
EPRDF	Ethiopian People's Revolutionary Democratic Front
HIV	human immunodeficiency virus
OLF	Oromo Liberation Front
TPLF	Tigray People's Liberation Front

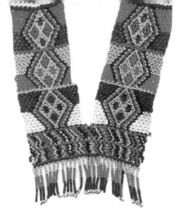

Preface

In and around the ancient trade center of Harar, Ethiopia, Oromo women live as traders, wood carriers, shepherds, and farmers. They have faced food scarcity, political conflict, the confiscation of their ancestral land, and severe restrictions on personal freedom. These same women, both young and old, adorn themselves with an array of body art. These forms of body art, including beaded jewelry, elaborate hairstyles, facial markings and particular dress, require great effort. On my first trip to Harar, I wondered why Oromo women, who often live below the poverty line in Ethiopia, spend so much time, money, and energy on decorating their bodies. This book is my attempt to answer this question.

By tracing the development of dress within the Oromo social system from the mid-nineteenth century to today, and through a close examination of dress activated on the body in particular contexts, the reader will uncover how truly valuable a woman's decorated body is as an aesthetic and symbolic system. Dress mirrors Oromo constructions of history and identity. To explore dress and the decorated body in history and cultural practice, this book examines past events that inform present-day choices in coiffure, jewelry, clothing, and skin markings. In particular, Oromo dress in relation to trade, the introduction to Islam, the disintegration of traditional Oromo institutions, and the political changes brought about by the conquest of Oromo lands by the Ethiopian Empire inform the first half of the text. The second half of this book focuses on the use of dress and the decorated body within Oromo cosmology, law, and lifecycle stages as a woman moves from childhood through old age. Art historical and anthropological approaches to dress are knit together through the complex and often contradictory ways that women think about and construct a sense of what it means to be Oromo. This includes choices around concealing versus revealing, and repelling versus attracting when they dress up.

This book, which is the first study of body art in Oromia, contributes to our understanding of Ethiopian culture and history, body art and performance, gender and identity, and African art history. By questioning how Oromo women have used historic experience, cultural knowledge, and body art as resources in formulating and displaying ethnic identity and historical consciousness, it elaborates on the path laid by some scholars who have focused their attention on the formation of nationalism and identity among traditionally peripheralized and underrepresented peoples of Ethiopia (Baxter; Hultin and Triulzi; Donham and James; Fukui and Markakis; Gebissa; Hassen; I. M. Lewis). It also highlights areas of Oromo cultural practice and performance that have been virtually ignored, despite their importance. This research bridges the gap between literature dedicated to male sociopolitical institutions, such as *gada*, in which generational grades are marked by what one wears (Baxter; Blackhurst; Hinnant; Legesse) and literature on female-dominated institutions such as spirit possession, which does not address the important role of art in possession performances (Braukamper; Gibb; Hecht; Hinnant; H. Lewis; Morton; Waldron). This text also contributes to the growing literature on Ethiopian art and challenges scholarship that categorizes arts of the body and arts of the non-Christian regions as merely 'craft' or 'material culture.' Published work on the art of Ethiopia consists largely of Orthodox Christian icons, church architecture, and religious paintings (Chojnacki; Gerster; Gnisci; Heldman; Mercier; Pankhurst; Perczel). While other scholarly attention has shifted to encompass the economic and political nature of non-Christian Ethiopia, the aesthetic expressions of many other groups, especially the Oromo, have yet to be thoroughly documented, analyzed and incorporated into Ethiopian art history.

Within African art history, this research combines and extends two key insights that produced critical orientations in the field but have rarely been joined. Body art, such as jewelry, has traditionally been studied as a static art in the discipline of art history. By drawing on R. F. Thompson's (1974) classic argument that African art must be seen in motion to be efficacious to participants and understood by scholars, this book views Oromo women's adornment in active contexts such as pilgrimages, spirit possession groups, and everyday life. Further, this study draws on, and contributes to, interdisciplinary writings on the clothed and decorated body that center on relations among fashion, identity, and gender (Arnoldi and Kreamer; Bann; Barnes; Bell; Eicher; Hendrickson; Hollander; Klumpp and Kratz; Roach-Higgins; Eicher and Johnson; Rovine), and performance studies in which historical change, political circumstances, and the resistance and acceptance of social norms are played out in ceremonial situations (e.g., M. Drewal; Hinnant; Kratz; Spencer; Turner). Can this study, then, remedy the absence of Oromo art and expressive culture in African art history? Of course not. It is only the beginning, with hopes that as Ethiopia continues to democratize and more scholars learn about Oromo arts, further research will flourish. By focusing intensively on one region of Oromia with subsequent trips to different areas, this research, first and foremost, introduces this salient form of Oromo art to a wider audience.

After two, short preliminary trips in 1996 and 1998, I undertook a year's study in 1999–2000 near the town of Harar situated in the Central Highlands of Ethiopia, and subsequent research trips in 2004, 2006 and 2010 in Wallo, Karrayyu, and the Arsi areas of the Oromia and Amhara regions of Ethiopia. I also conducted archival research for four months at the Institute of Ethiopian Studies, Addis Ababa University. While at the Institute, I documented the costume repertoire in the institute's museum, and gathered information and visual images from their archives on patterns of use, changes in meaning, and styles of wear of traditional Oromo dress. In 2006 and 2010, I also spent time in Nairobi, Kenya, specifically in the East Leigh neighborhood where many Oromo refugees from Ethiopia reside today and dress largely to disguise their Oromo identity. Since 2016, I have been working with the Oromo Diaspora in the United States and Canada. In each place, I was interested in locating the form, function, and meaning of objects of adornment that communicated distinct stories about what it means to be Oromo. These stories were often connected to oral accounts collected over many hours in my home outside the walled city of Harar. I shared this home with my research associate, Bakkalcha Yaya, who, as a poet and former songwriter for the then outlawed Oromo Liberation Front (OLF), needed to remain hidden. His encyclopedic knowledge of Oromo cultural practice, genealogy, and ritual helped to guide our daily interviews and he could quickly tell what valuable knowledge each individual could offer this study. Since there was no extensive historical framework in place for this region of Oromia, I began by asking very basic questions about the connections between dress and historical experiences. As my research associate's travel ability was limited, we would often invite knowledgeable folks from the countryside for lunch and a *khat* chewing session, followed by taped interviews that lasted until the sunset prayer. Then my research associate and I would continue late into the night with transcriptions.[1]

With the assistance of the Oromo Culture and Information Bureau, I also secured permission to record ceremonies and conduct interviews in a dozen towns in the surrounding countryside. Slowly, I began to realize what was important to record for the Oromo community. This study is a collection of our melded voices.

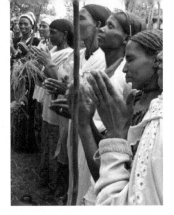

Acknowledgements

In Harar, I extend my sincere appreciation to the many Oromo research associates who contributed to this project. Some of their names appear in abbreviated form in the bibliography but there are dozens more whom I can only inadequately thank here with a collective word of gratitude. The research scholars at the East Hararghe Orominya Culture and Information Office, the Oromo Regional Bureau in Jarso and Baabile, and the Somali Bureau in Baabile generously provided their time and resources to make this study a success. My deepest gratitude goes to the numerous individuals who have assisted this research by offering their time, knowledge, hospitality, and friendship: Ahmed Zekaria, Zewdu Gebreweld, Sirag Ahmed, Mustafa Abbas Tosha, Abdullahi Ali Sherif, Adam Sherif, Sala Hadin, Guutamma Ammallee, Taman Youssoff, Guluma Gemeda, Asfaw Beyene, Habtamu Dugo, Nina and Janet Redwan, and Mohammednoor Ahmed Toyib and his family. I would also like to thank the museum staff at the Institute of Ethiopian Studies who patiently assisted me in locating and photographing objects, and in the installation of my exhibition *Women's Costumes in Eastern Ethiopia* sponsored by the U.S. Embassy in 2000 and *Bareedina: Women of Oromia* in 2011. I am also indebted to fellow researcher Bedri Kabir who helped me to formulate this project in 1998 and whose crucial work on the history of the Afran Qallo Oromo served as an important framework for the first half of this book. Two individuals in particular, Bakkalcha Yaya and Iftu Mahammed, who become in the course of my stay in Ethiopia the brother and sister I have always wanted, deserve special recognition. Bakkalcha's immense knowledge and gentle tolerance will always be remembered. As primary research collaborator, every section of this book is infused with his *ayyanna*. I also acknowledge the memories of Ahmed and Fatuma, whom I lost during my stay in Harar but whose voices live on in the following pages.

In 2010, the Oromia Culture and Tourism Bureau in Addis Ababa graciously sponsored my project, provided photographs, and offered field assistance. I particularly wish to thank Daniel Deressa, Sintayehu Tola, and Belay Kassayye. In Bati, Abdulkader Mohammed and Jemal Adem from the Bati Bureau of Culture and Tourism were very helpful, and in Kemise, Ahamd Sa'eed from the Kamise

Culture and Tourism Office and O. Sayid at the Oromia Zone Culture and Tourism Bureau, Amhara Region, provided cultural objects to photograph. In Arsi, the late Boonsamoo Mi'eessoo of the West Arsi Zone Center and Tourism Office shared his important research on women's dress with enthusiasm. This trip would not have been fruitful without the expert guidance of Mohammedtahir Abduselam Aliyi during trips to Wallo in 2010 and the kindness of his family in Kemise.

I am indebted to Dr. Mohammed Hassen, Emeritus Professor, in the Department of History at Georgia State University, whose research on the Oromo has most significantly informed my understanding of Oromo history and, in turn, has cultivated my compassion for all people living under conditions of subordination. His belief in me and tireless readings of drafts made this publication possible. I graciously thank and remember my late advisor Dr. Sidney Kasfir at Emory University who served as the first reader of this text. Her important work on masking, spirit possession, and contemporary African art has significantly shaped both what and how I study. Over a decade later, scholar and social activist Bonnie Holcomb (Qabbanee), was the last to read my manuscript. Her unyielding efforts on behalf of the Oromo people and her scholarship on Oromo identity have my deepest admiration.

I am also grateful for the scholarly engagement with the following mentors and colleagues who helped shape the theoretical and methodological ideas for the initial fieldwork and early writings: Corrine Kratz, the late Ivan Karp, Mike McGovern, Raymond Silverman, Neal Sobania, Donald Donham, Sunanda Sanyal, Jessica Stephenson, Krista Thompson, Jeremy Pool, Jay Straker, Leah Niederstadt, and Obse Ababiya.

I'd also like to thank the talented Yadesa Bojia for his beautiful painting for the book cover and Yasin Ib, Tunsia Mohammed, Harar Photo Studio, and Mickey Photography for the use of their images. I am grateful for editorial help from Dina Ormenyi, Diana Coetze and Zakia Posey and my gracious editor, Kassahun Checole of Africa World Press, who has brought a dizzying number of valuable books on Africa to life.

This book would not be possible without research support. I would like to wholeheartedly thank the J. William Fulbright Scholarship Board for granting me the Fulbright Fellowship for my first field research (1999–2000), the Internationalization Research Fellowship from Emory University for financial assistance (2000, 2002), and the Mike Curb College of Arts, Media, and Communication and the Art Department at California State University, Northridge for research and publication support (2010, 2015, 2019).

My two lovely daughters have waited their whole lives for this book to be finished. May they be inspired to travel, study, and work in Africa. Finally, to all Afran Qallo Oromo whose art and history are recorded in these pages, this book is for you.

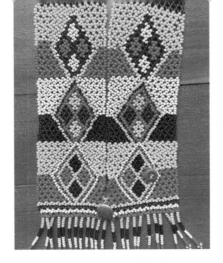

Chapter One:

Introduction:
Dress and the Decorated Female Body in Oromia

"my mother was my first country. the first place i ever lived."

—nayyirah waheed

Fatuma, an Oromo refugee, shrouded in black, steps nimbly over rotting trash in the soupy mud, dodging the spray of city buses. She is disguised as a Somali woman in black hijab, donning the sanctioned garb of the al-Shabab mosques. Her dress is an attempt to hide from Kenyan gang members, Kenyan police, Somalis, and others hostile to the growing refugee population in and around Nairobi but, most importantly, to keep Ethiopian government scouts whose job it is to hunt those accused of terrorism at bay. These scouts, dressed in civilian clothing and operating with full authorization of the Kenyan government, take refugees by force back to Addis Ababa, the Ethiopian capital, to stand trial. Fatuma knows from experience that most trials result in lifetime incarceration, torture, rape, and death. She, like many of the Oromo refugees from Ethiopia living in the slums outside Nairobi or in Dadaab or Kakuma refugee camp, are corporeally aware of their Oromo identity – they wear it proudly in certain circumstances and go to great length to disguise it in others.

Thousands of miles to the north at the Ethnographic Museum of the Institute of Ethiopian Studies on the Addis Ababa University campus, hundreds of hair combs, headrests, silver amulets, beaded jewelry, baskets, musical instruments, and sacred objects of the Oromo are proudly on display for schoolchildren, foreign visitors, and university students. Yet Oromo youth, despite their majority in number within Ethiopia, are scarce on campus. Thoughtfully curated vitrines of Oromo material culture are lavishly exhibited, but very few Oromo ever see them. The objects are situated there to promote an Ethiopian national heritage, but with little thought to the people themselves.[2] In North America, Oromo at a Los Angeles reservoir gather annually to celebrate Irreechaa, a thanksgiving ritual honoring the Oromo supreme being, Waqaa. In a sea of white clothing emblazoned with images of the sycamore tree fresh grasses in hand, they make their way to a large pond in a public park to pray as joggers and picnickers turn their heads to watch. Whether in Oromia, Ethiopia; in transit in the waystations of places such as Nairobi and Djibouti; or in the ever-growing migrant communities of the Oromo Diaspora, dress becomes strategically worn.

This book centers on Oromo women's body art and cultural practices. Within Ethiopia, Oromo women have lived with the uncertainties of drought, war, political unrest, food shortage, land scarcity, and personal insecurity for several generations. They have experienced growing poverty, disease, and rapid land loss under villagization policies of the Military Regime (1974–1991) and, more recently, under the Ethiopian People's Revolutionary Democratic Front (EPRDF) policies of the Master Plan, forcibly implemented between 2014 and 2018, which led to hundreds of thousands of Oromo farmers' removal from their ancestral land. These same women, both young and old, adorn themselves with a rich repertoire of body art. Jewelry articulates arms, fingers, necks, and ears. Faces are enhanced with subtle scars and tattoos. Hair is plaited and dressed in hairnets and scarves. The body is wrapped in layers of white sheeting or colorful textiles. An Oromo woman's decorated body is layered with intended messages that communicate her personal experiences, represent and reproduce her position in society, impart information about her political and spiritual beliefs, and visually indicate her Oromo identity. Through the lens of dress, this book gives voice to moments in the complex history of one of the largest ethnic groups in Africa who has undergone radical socio-political changes in the nineteenth and twentieth centuries in an important crossroads region of the world.

My interest in Oromo women's dress began in the ancient walled city of Harar in Eastern Ethiopia in 1998 when I first observed the ensemble of dress worn by Oromo wood sellers, who are among the poorest laborers in Ethiopia. As Ethiopia is almost completely deforested, women will spend several days collecting enough kindling to bundle and sell for a day's worth of legumes and grain. Ignorant of the communicative capacity of their dress, I was nonetheless amazed at women's investment in personal adornment, including costumes made from leather, metal, wood, amber, bone, horn, shells, plastic beads, and imported cloth. The Oromo constitute the ethnic majority within Ethiopia, but they have historically been marginalized politically, economically, and socially within the Ethiopian state. They have lived under Ethiopian imperial rule most of the last century and under intermittent conditions of subordination since the conquest and incorporation of the region of Hararghe into the expanding Ethiopian empire in 1887. I began to wonder why women who were so economically disadvantaged spent so much time, energy, and resources on their personal appearance.

During a trip to the city of Dire Dawa in 2000, I interviewed a group of older Oromo men and a few women in a private compound outside the city center. It was one of the first group interviews I conducted while in residency in Harar. After waiting months in the capital for research clearance, I worried that my project would not have much relevance and value to these elders. They had spent the morning counseling a community of farmers who lacked adequate water, who had recently lost half their harvest, and who relied heavily on foreign grain rations that were slow in coming. Half serious, farmers told us: "When we are hungry, we pray for rain in Canada." Showering male elders with inquiries about women's dress and cultural practices felt, during this first interview, intrusive and frivolous. As I passed around photographs, my research associate and I began asking my long list of prepared questions late into the afternoon. Our host's cousin found a small boy to buy more *khat* (also *qat*) and Coke in hopes of sweeting my barrage of inquiries. At the end of the session, as we prepared to go, three men asked that we allow them to record messages on my cassette recorder. It illustrates to some extent the weight that I came to understand Oromo dress carries, especially at moments of crisis, and especially when one's identity is under fire:

> We want to send a message to the Americans who might read your book. The government has barred our history many times and people who have tried to learn our history have been killed time and time again. We are happy that you want to know our history. It is time that it is brought out from the place where it is buried and shared with the world. We have been asked by the rulers of Ethiopia to hide our identity and we were afraid to say we were Oromo. Still, now we cannot explain much because we cannot speak freely. Can you believe that we reached this standard? When a man wears his *fila* (wooden hair comb) and a woman her cultural dress, they must be careful since others may relate it to political involvement. They may be killed or imprisoned. But they must do so. Do you understand? Otherwise, we are no better off than those who were killed or arrested. We pray that our conditions will improve. (I.A., February 20, 2000)

A study of Oromo women's dress and their decorated bodies (and, to a lesser extent, men's adornment) in Eastern Ethiopia, I quickly learned, could offer a rich portrait of what it means to be part of the great nation of Oromia. Expressly the decorated female body, rooted firmly in a collective historical trajectory and an indigenous aesthetic system, has much to tell us about how people make sense of their world and signal their shared experiences. By examining specific body modifications and supplements, I found that a fundamental dialectic exists among dress, the female body, and the ways in which Barentuma Oromo actively assemble projections of themselves. Whether Muslim, Christian, traditional practitioner, semi-nomadic herder or sedentary agriculturalist, Oromo throughout Oromia use dress to signify Oromummaa (Oromoness).

The Oromo in Eastern Oromia

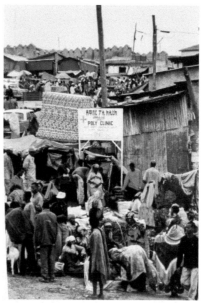

Figure 1.1   Harar Market

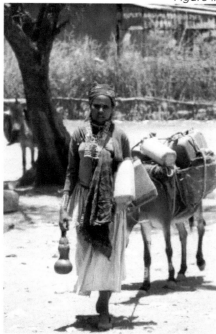

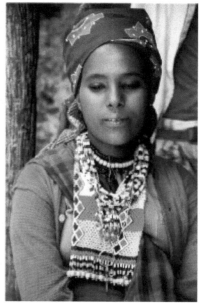

Figure 1.2 Oromo Kerosene Seller in Baabile Town headed to Harar

On any given day, the main thoroughfare in the city of Harar in Eastern Oromia is usually crowded, with long lines of pedestrians weaving back and forth amidst taxis, domestic animals, and vendors (Figure 1.1). Oromo women burdened with donkeys and bundles of wood on their heads make their way to and from the main market. They are clearly distinct: a dress of *abu jedid* factory cloth ending at mid-calf belted with an imported sash, wide necklaces and headbands of colorful seed beads, an old sash with which to secure small children or merchandise on their backs, and a tight-fitting, striped T-shirt made in China (Figure 1.2). Neighboring Harari women pass draped in shiny sumptuous head scarves wearing pleated pastel dresses that reveal finely embroidered pants underneath. Somali women conceal their bodies and hair in wide Indian gauzes of crimson and tangerine that they hold together on windy days with black henna-stained hands covered in locally made gold rings.

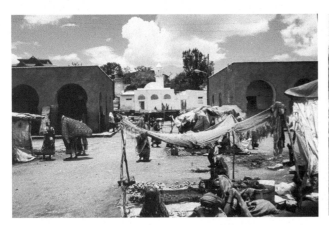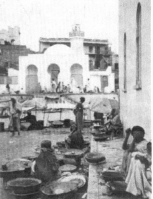

Figure 1.3 Oromo Vegetable Vendors in Harar in the early 2000's and the early 1960's (Second Source: Burton 1967, 92)

All groups, including the Muslim Argobba and Christian Amhara, make use of imported textiles and accessories found in the Harar market, nicknamed 'Taiwan,' where contraband electronic and clothing merchandise are smuggled from ports in Djibouti. Many of these same articles become incorporated into costumes across ethnic lines. For example, the white cotton cloth used by Oromo women for their dresses is also worn by Somali women (Figure 1.4); an Oromo married woman's black hairnet is like that of an Argobba woman (Figure 1.5); and the metal forehead ornaments worn by young Oromo and Harari women differ only in material (Figure 1.6). Yet, each ethnic dress ensemble is clearly distinct. Women make specific choices in dress based on a whole host of issues, but, above all, they choose materials and styles of wear that are culturally appropriate. While Harari women wear nail polish on their nails, for example, Oromo women prefer to dab polish on their cheeks in patterns that mimic older and more permanent tattoo practices (Figure 1.7).

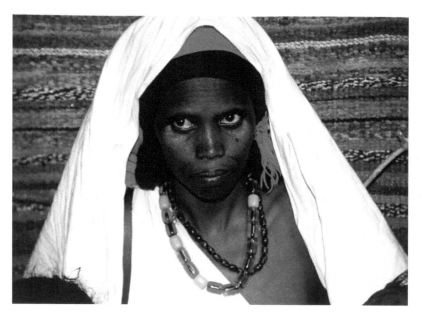

Figure 1.4 A Somali Woman wearing White Sheeting and Imitation Amber

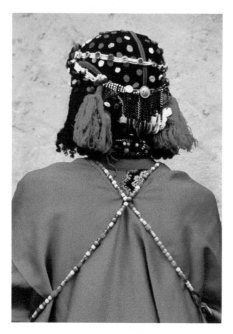

Figure 1.5 An Argobba Woman with Mesh Hairnet Ornamented with Embroidery and Headbands

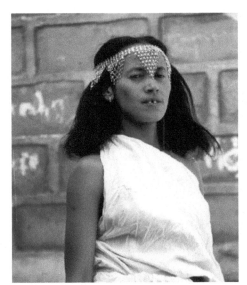 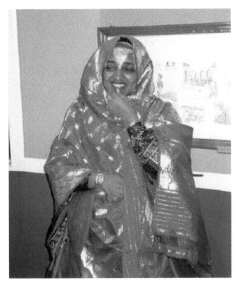

Figure 1.6 (Left) An Oromo Woman's Silver Headband, Qarmaa Loti
(Right) A Harari Woman's Gold Headband, Siyassa

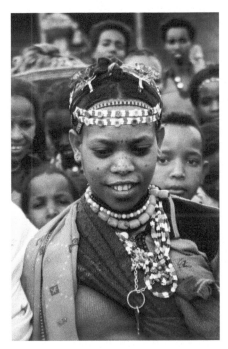

Figure 1.7 A Young Afran Qallo Woman with
Beaded Adornment and Kula Facial Markings

The Oromo who reside in Ethiopia are organized into lineages and adorn themselves with a great variety of dress styles and forms. I will only address a few. I have also limited my geographic parameters to the Barentuma Oromo, one half of the great Oromo Confederacy.[3] The Barentuma are themselves a diverse and vast group, and this study addresses cultural practices in only a handful of regions. I began the first six months of fieldwork collecting information on genealogy, politics, religion, cosmology, astronomy, lifecycle rituals, divination, and gender before moving to a detailed discussion of dress. Despite the fact that the Oromo are one of the largest ethnic groups in Africa (35–40 million) and their language is the third most widely spoken on the continent, in-depth studies on the Barentuma, in general, are lacking and for any understanding of aesthetics and dress, greatly needed.[4] The absence of information on the opulent artforms and performances of the Oromo in contrast to the strong scholarship on the material heritage of the Orthodox Christian Church in Ethiopia says a great deal about restricted access by scholars, academic surveillance, and the tumultuous relationship of the Oromo within the Ethiopian regime. The fact remains that after the forced exile of foreign academics during the Marxist regime in the 1970s and 1980s, many have chosen not to return (for fear of their safety and that of their families in returning) since the reopening of the country to outside scholars in the early 1990s. Furthermore, owing to the volatility of the political situation, many scholars of the Oromo in the Diaspora felt that they were at personal risk if they returned. It is in this climate that I began my own inquiries about dress, representation and political consciousness.[5]

My fieldwork relied heavily on important texts devoted to Oromo cultural and socio-political institutions, the development of Oromo consciousness, and the Oromo experience within the Ethiopian Empire (Baxter, Hultin, and Triulzi 1994; Donham and James 1986; Freeman and Pankhurst 2003; Fukui and Markakis 1994; Gebissa 2009; Hassen 2017; Holcomb and Ibssa 1990; I.M. Lewis 1983; Jalata 2007, 2005, 1998). Yet, this work has paid little attention to related Oromo artistic manifestations. By examining how Oromo women have used their shared cultural knowledge to decorate their bodies, this book expands the socio-historical path laid by these scholars by including the important role that women's agency and art play in the construction of identity and the formulation of historical consciousness. Since Oromo identity has been principally equated with male identity, this study of Oromo women and their arts not only presents a fuller picture of the construction of Oromo identity, but also presents a new understanding of how women represent themselves and are represented.

This book is divided into two parts. The first half examines the ways events in the Oromo past that have precipitated political, economic, and social changes have become conceptually embedded in certain kinds of jewelry, clothing, hairdressings, and skin markings. These historical instances include the introduction of Islam to the Barentuma Oromo, their participation in historical trade routes, the disintegration of their indigenous institutions, and the political changes brought about by the incorporation of the Oromo into the Ethiopian Empire. These events span roughly two hundred years or seven generations, and include other players whose material, expressive and religious culture have affected, and at times dominated, Oromo dress: the Harari, Argobba, Amhara, Egyptian, Somali, and Tigre.

The second half of this book focuses more closely on the use of dress and the decorated body within significant social contexts in women's lives, including spirit possession, lifecycle rituals, and ideas about the female body within Oromo law. In thinking about how to structure this section, I looked to Perani and Wolff (1999, 29) who discuss the ways in which dress has "overlapping mediating functions" such as a signifier of spiritual belief, a way to define and negotiate power, and a marker of cultural change. In both the broad, historical overview and the more specific, body-centered investigation of dress, several diametrically opposed tensions resurface in the meanings of various body art practices. These include concealing versus revealing, repelling versus attracting, beautifying versus disfiguring, tying versus cutting, and, to a lesser extent, dryness versus wetness/shininess. It is my intention that these ideas function as conceptual threads that bind the two analytical approaches in writing together. The book ends with a discussion of fashion and locality within contemporary nationalist discourse.

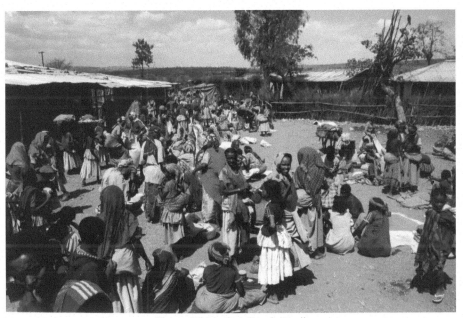

Figure 1.8 Market Day in Fedis

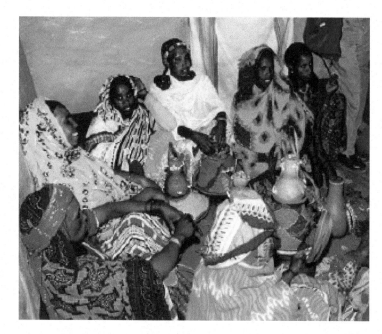

Figure 1.9 Afran Qallo Women engaged in Wadaajaa Prayer Ceremony

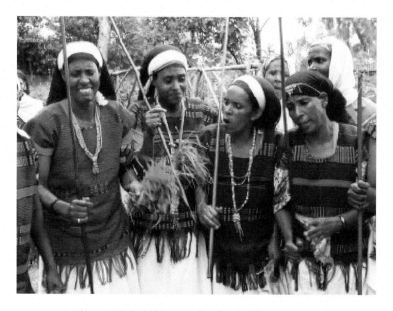

Figure 1.10 Arsi Women singing in Shashamene

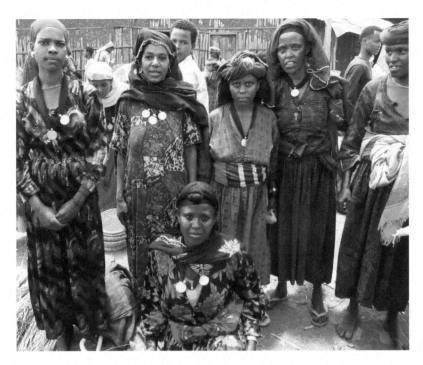

Figure 1.11 Wallo Women shopping for Ingredients for the Ceremonial Smoke Bath, Qayyaa in Kemise

The Oromo within the Discourse on Dress

Austrian ethnographer Philip Paulitschke (1888a, 52), who visited Ethiopia in the 1880s, described Oromo women's adornment as a "conceptual system." The Oromo aesthetic of dress arrangement is dependent on two competing concepts within Oromo society. On the one hand, sacred objects and acts should be kept hidden. In this sense, the most spiritually or socially powerful body art practices should not be perceptibly pronounced. On the other hand, women should be recognized first and foremost for their ethnic distinction; a process that is only possible by drawing attention to the ensemble of things with which they decorated their bodies.

In Rugh's (1986, 54) study of contemporary Egyptian dress where I first came across this notion of revealing versus concealing, she writes: "rural woman, even with choice of style severely limited . . . may wonder whether to identify her origins by known markers in an unfamiliar place . . . or to walk anonymously among strangers, saving the more subtle signs she wishes to communicate to members of the inner circle."

These two ideals between hiding that which is most value-laden and making available the visual symbols of Oromo identity are brought into dialogue on the body through an aesthetic of accumulation.[6] This accumulation of body modifications and supplements is mapped together onto the body creating a layering of form, color, and texture to the eye achieved at a woman's head, for example, by layering fiber, cloth, and beaded bands over and under a hairnet and headscarf. The head may be further ornamented with flowers and herb sprigs, while more potent medicines and stones remain tucked up and hidden under the hair. This layering effect both disguises the clarity of individual objects and brings them into a relational patterning with other similar and different items. As objects shift in position or as they are replaced with items of more modern appeal, such as plastic beads and suede over glass beads and leather, they continue to be arranged through this accumulated aesthetic (Figure 1.12).

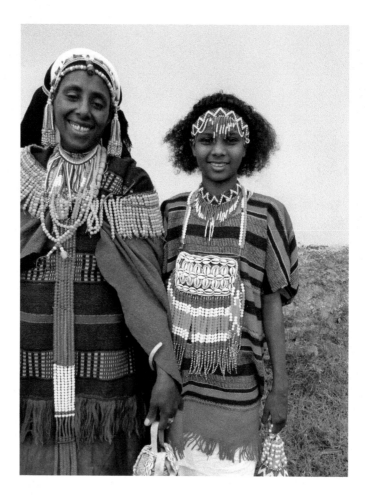

Figure 1.12 Contemporary Arsi Dress

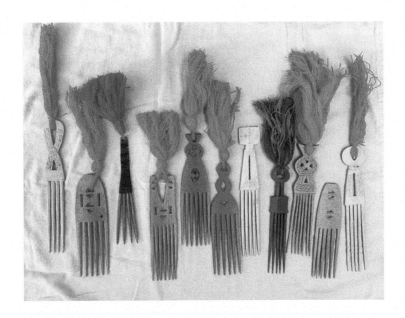

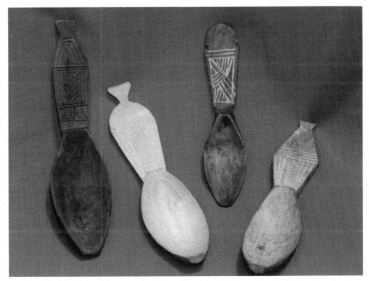

Figure 1.13 Oromo Carved Combs fashioned for Men's Hair
Figure 1.14 Oromo Carved Spoons

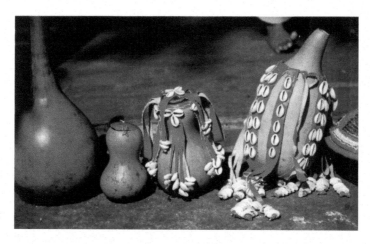

Figure 1.15 Oromo Gourds ornamented with Vinyl and Cowrie Shells

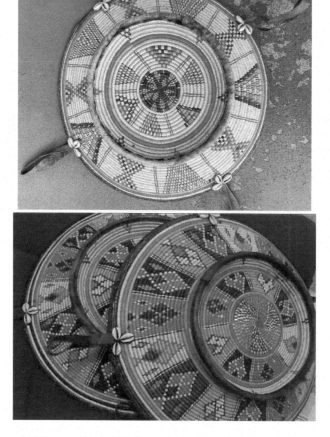

Figure 1.16 Oromo Baskets influenced by Harari Shape and Materials

The variety and mass of material that has come to define the Oromo aesthetic is not, however, dependent upon localized production. While some aspects of dress are clearly Oromo-made, such as the beaded necklaces and the elaborate hairstyles, many objects are also produced in factories in the commercial town of Dire Dawa or overseas. While a limited male carving tradition exists in the production of wooden hair combs, and wooden spoons, and etched gourds with non-figural, geometric designs (Figure 1.13, 1.14, 1.15), there are no professional women's groups who produce personal arts. Among the neighboring Harari, however, a basket-making co-operative has been in existence in the Harari Cultural Center since 1999. This group of roughly two dozen women plait baskets in a large, public room in the house of the late French poet Rimbaud, now a cultural heritage site. Their products are sold in the Rimbaud gift shop. Among the Oromo, there is, as yet, little market for their beadwork or baskets. Their baskets, based on Harari forms, are uniquely Oromo in design (Figure 1.16). Women create baskets and dress sets in their free time without formal apprenticeship, and with the resources at their disposal, often including imported items and materials.

Oromo women certainly participate in active and passive types of artistic evaluation, including, in the case of beadwork, purchasing and stringing the beads, scrutinizing the tedious hand movements of advanced beaders, participating in beading groups, and analyzing and criticizing the finished products of expert beaders. Because dress, like other personal art objects, should remain within prescribed Oromo artistic boundaries, and because no great value is placed on innovation in and of itself, women would be harshly criticized by peers and female relations if they strayed into great degrees of innovation. Unless there are external influences such as new techniques and materials that can easily translate into Oromo artistic codes, clothing, adornment, and facial markings are resistant to the rapid shifts of fashion.

In their discussion of ornaments among the Booran Oromo, Kassam and Megersa (1989, 23) point out the difficulty in direct semantic translation between Oromo and Euro-American notions of adornment. Oromo describe jewelry in particular as *nagata* (putting on), *waan fayya* (beautiful things) or, more rarely, *mard'aad* (that which goes round). An object worn on the body is as much noted for the act of its placement and for the relationship it holds to the body and other objects as for its ability to beautify. For this reason, body modifications and supplements are examined not only in relation to other body art practices, but also in relation to the body, especially the body as it is socially and physically located within Oromo society. As Entwistle (2001, 37) mentions: "dress lies at the margins of the body and marks the boundary between self and other, individual and society." Dress is therefore a culturally present second skin that may favor certain kinds of identities, both for the self and for the larger community. The way in which abstract principles such as moral codes and ethnic affiliations become embedded in, and communicated through, tangible forms is a complex negotiation. As objects and bodies change through time and place, meaning also fluctuates and shifts. Some types of adornment, such as coins, for example, are used by women to arrest destructive power transferred through the gaze, reflect the evil eye and ward off spiritual attacks. Once afflicted or possessed by a *jarrii* spirit, however, young women might wear coins in accordance with their spirit's demands. Young women also wear coins to sparkle and attract the attention of potential suitors. To tease out how dress becomes meaningful to the Oromo, I will bring into dialogue a dense set of ideas and a range of object types. While the personal arts selected are each distinct in form, material, placement on the body, and significance, I will demonstrate that each is conceptually rooted in the Oromo aesthetic system.

Dress as a tactical means of asserting a political identity, empowering formerly subjugated people, and challenging the power of a regime has been excellently documented in several African cultures (Hendrickson 1996; Allman 2004) and, specifically among Muslim women (Becker 2006; Renne 2013). Rugh's (1986) work among Muslim Egyptian women in particular demonstrates that dress is the most significant strategy women have for asserting meaning. The dressed and decorated body is herein considered as an aesthetic and symbolic system with which women tactically prioritize and communicate social beliefs and values.

All bodily alterations to be examined fall under the rubric of dress, defined by Eicher and Roach-Higgins (1992, 15) as "an assemblage of body modifications and/or supplements displayed by a person in communicating with other human beings." "Dress," as expressed by Arthur (1999, 7), "provides a window through which we might look into a culture, because it visually attests to the salient ideas, concepts and categories fundamental to that culture." I will use the terms 'dress', 'adornment', and 'costume' interchangeably in this text to suggest the ensemble of arts that embellish or alter the body. As such, costume may include permanent genres such as tattooing and scarification, as well as semi or non-permanent decorations such as henna and clothing. When assembled on the body, this repertory of adornment shapes the projection of self, social values, and social structures. 'Costume', after all, is historically derived from 'custom.' Both terms indicate that material culture and social forms are used contextually to construct identities through the medium of social relations.

Dress, Gender, and Change

Ethnography that focuses on only one sex is problematic. Beidelman (1997, 24) correctly asserts that "the definition and implications of male gender cannot be separated from those of female gender, and both pose challenges to analytical revision." Since this project focuses almost exclusively on women's body art, an explanation for this topic is essential.

A gendered politics of dress is typically found in all societies. In her examination of gender and fashion, Entwistle (2000, 143) states that "clothing, as an aspect of culture, is a crucial feature in the production of masculinity and femininity; it turns nature into culture, layering cultural meanings on the body." The tendency for men to wear modern dress, for example, while traditional styles are reserved for women is consistent throughout most of the Horn of Africa and the Middle East. Lindisfarne-

Tapper and Ingham (1997, 28) attribute this phenomenon to the creation of gender models by centralized states that regulate men through duties such as military service and trade. They write: "It is much more likely that women's dress, by default or choice, signals identities which are forbidden or precluded to men" (129). Similarly, Wood (1999, 41) asserts that among the Gabra Oromo in Kenya, men opt for dress that they perceive as urban and modern, while women's dress in both urban and rural situations is always visibly Gabra. This binary association of women with the domestic realm and men with the public sphere in non-Western societies has been explained in feminist thought as a form of patriarchal control. Since women are associated with childbearing and domesticity in society, they cannot fully participate in the public arena and socio-political organizations dominated by men (Rosaldo 1974, 23–24; Ortner 1974, 77–79). Among the Barentuma Oromo, dress also falls into these gendered spaces and gendered domains, since women tend to be associated with cultural dress and domesticity, and men with more "modern" attire and the public realm. The restrictions placed on women's bodies in public spaces, particularly the covering of the head through Islamic prescription, has become an important convention. Yet, the role of most female dress types is largely excluded from this discourse of male control, especially since the same sets of adornment are worn in various social and spatial contexts. Among the Oromo, it is women's dressed bodies (in typically more insular spaces less open to the scrutiny of non-Oromo) that become vehicles for expressions of ethnonational affiliations. Owing to men's more active participation in state-sponsored organizations, they are more likely to be harassed through the bodily display of objects prescribed by the government to promote "narrow nationalism." While men's dress is selectively discussed in this book, it is largely not the focus because it is not directly relevant to the perpetuation of an Oromo identity in Oromia. This is somewhat different than the current situation in the Diaspora, where there has been a profusion of men's shirts and pants emblazoned with the Oromo flag.

Oromo men in Oromia today don Western-style pants or waist wrappers from Indonesia, long-sleeved button shirts or polyester T-shirts from China, and a variety of second-hand clothing from Europe, Canada, and the United States like their Amhara, Afar, Argobba, Harari, Somali, and Tigre male neighbors from whom they are virtually indistinguishable. This homogenous look is due, in part, to men's access to public spheres and long-distance travel, through their engagement in activities such as trading, cattle herding and working communal farms, and through Islamic pilgrimage. Further, time spent wearing specialized uniforms while in the military or while imprisoned in jail or underground detention centers, has psychologically conditioned men to a homogenized look. On another level this bodily sameness may serve as a screen that Oromo men can use to filter out markers of Oromo culture from non-Oromo public scrutiny. Oromo women, however, appear distinct, often rejecting materials and designs that seem too "foreign" or styles that had been co-opted by other local ethnicities. Women's decorated bodies function as discrete markers of ethnic expression in contrast and often in opposition to the adorned bodies of men. Men's participation in the evaluation of this material, however, is extremely important. Since older men act as household and village representatives, many of those interviewed about dress for this project were, in fact, men. Therefore, while the focus of this text is centered on women's personal arts, it is the messages that these arts convey to both men and women in the community that are crucial to my analysis.

With the constant influx of new materials into the markets today, coupled with ongoing instability from events such as famine, military clashes, and historic fighting between the ruling party and Oromo civilians, it is certain that many types of body art are reconfigured in form and given new layers of meaning by current events. During the famines in the early 2000s, for example, many Oromo and Somali women near Harar sold their most valuable silver jewelry and amber necklaces to Harari families.[7] Harari women began to sell them to outsiders. As tourism is seasonal and today rather sparse, the four Harari boutiques active during the time of my fieldwork were located in the sitting rooms of private compounds within the city. While this jewelry could be loaned out to Oromo locals for special occasions until tourists bought them, most Oromo women were leery of these contracts and resorted, instead, to using imitation amber and industrial metal or tin for their costumes. I could only find a handful of Oromo woman who still owned real amber or resin beads, and silver filigree hair ornaments. Clearly, personal objects are by no means fixed markers of what it means to be Oromo in the modern era, which is why they may hold appeal to others, like me, who study dress and fashion – their style, meaning, and materials are dynamic.

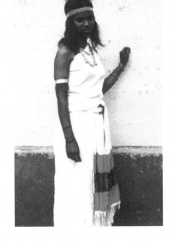

Chapter Two:

Fashioning History, Memory, and Meaning in Harar

We used to say that we hide our identity in the *gaadii*, the leather strap that ties the cow's back legs when milking. This kept our identity hidden to the foreigners that came and tried to destroy it. Nowadays, our traditions are privately articulated through women's *hibboo* (songs), *ufata* (dressing), and *hellee* (dancing). Since many of our young men and [male] elders were killed by the Turks and, later, the Abyssinians, it is up to the women to carry along our *adaa* (culture). (M.S.S. March 1, 2000)

A sixty-three-year-old Afran Qallo Oromo man, himself a respected elder and spokesperson for his community, spoke these words. His telling remarks reveal the central themes of Oromo identity. As foreign powers threatened and continue to hinder Oromo practice, cultural expressions are kept safe through secrecy and their relegation to the more private domain of women. The leather strap tied to the back leg of the milking cow, for example, became the ideal identity idiom not only because it encompasses this notion of concealment, but it is made of leather, the central material for an Oromo women's traditional costume. The speaker echoes a sentiment that resonates throughout his community: women, as performers, educators, and icons are the carriers of cultural history through their decorated and performative bodies.

When the man quoted above learned I was collecting oral accounts of Oromo history, he came to speak with me in my home in Harar about Oromo genealogy. He spoke for five hours, recounting first the names of his forefathers some forty generations back, and then the line of descent of the Alla segmentary lineage (*gosa*) of the Afran Qallo. I listened with some apprehension since I had, at first, no intentions of collecting genealogies and creating kinship charts, and I had already limited my project to the parameters of three or four generations past – the length of time about which I thought most people could easily recollect and discuss. I often found throughout my fieldwork, however, that what my Oromo colleagues remembered as significant in the history of women's dress extended back several generations. Men and women remember their ancestry in order to navigate their present and future familial, legal, political, and social relationships. In the course of my discussions with people, the distant past was often more important to their sense of themselves as Oromo than the defining events that took place during the time of living relatives. Thereafter, I asked Afran Qallo Oromo elders to select significant historical moments, particularly accounts centered on genealogy, trade, and confrontations with outsiders that have most closely shaped women's dress within and around the city-state of Harar. Most men and women chose roughly the following three periods: (1) The Oromo migration to the Central Highlands, (2) the cloth trade and political dynamics between the Oromo and their neighbors during the last rulers of the Emirate of Harar (1850–1875), and (3) the Egyptian Occupation of Harar (1875–1885). Informants spoke freely about women's personal arts as they related to each of these periods and, by and large, the dress types most often mentioned include the classic Oromo dress of white sheeting, the sash that holds this dress in place, and silver filigree bracelets. These objects, still worn today, carry collective, historical memories that visually support oral accounts about who the Oromo are and where they came from.[8]

The Afran Qallo Oromo who live in and near the walled city of Harar exemplify some of the common experiences of all Barentuma Oromo, including contact, conquest, and colonization. As the previous quote by the Oromo elder states, it is moments of specific adversarial association with "Turks and Abyssinians" that threatened internal cohesion or created group fragmentation that have most dramatically influenced the symbolic significance and formal choices of adornment.

A Brief Introduction to the Oromo

The Oromo make up about forty percent of the population of Ethiopia, and also reside in western Somalia, northern Kenya and abroad. Within Ethiopia, the Oromo nation in Oromia reaches some 232,000 square miles from the Nile River in the north to the Hararghe Plateau in the southeast (Figure 2.1). The Oromia National Regional State makes up about thirty-five percent of the total land area of Ethiopia with 18 administrative zones. The area is rich in fertile land, water resources, mineral deposits, and forests. Many Oromo communities exist beyond the borders of Oromia, including the Wallo featured in this book. The current boundaries for the Oromia Regional State were established in 1992.

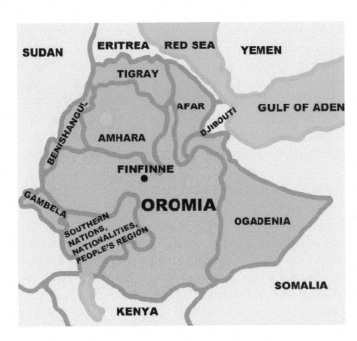

2.1 Map of Oromia

All Oromo speak a Cushitic language called 'Afaan Oromo' which, after Arabic and Hausa, is the most extensively used language on the African continent. Despite its widespread use, the Oromo language was only formally recognized and taught in schools during Ethiopia's brief Italian Occupation (1936–1941), and only under the present government has any significant progress been made in the development of the Oromo language on the national level, including the publication of the first texts exclusively in Afaan Oromo.[9]

When and from where the Oromo first appeared in present-day Ethiopia is a contentious issue that precipitates controversy about land use and indigeneity, and continues to be heavily debated among Oromo and non-Oromo populations alike. Most Ethiopianist scholarship characterizes Oromo movement into Ethiopia as a single wave of migration from either the Somali coast in the east, Lake Turkana in the south, or the Northern Highlands near present-day Bale spurred by pressures from Somali herders during the sixteenth century. These accounts rely heavily on a very biased and propagandistic account written by a monk named Bahrey who lived in southern Ethiopia. Bahrey (1993, 44), who wrote a history of the Oromo in 1593, states that his purpose for writing his text is "to make known the number of their tribe, their readiness to kill people and the brutality of their manner." More recent revisionist scholarship challenges the claim that the Oromo arrived en masse in the Ethiopian interior from somewhere outside its current boundaries, and that the Oromo migration and their subsequent assimilation was, in fact, a gradual transition that happened at different moments in different places. For example, Mohammed

Hassen (2017) has demonstrated an Oromo presence in the medieval Christian kingdom in the fourteenth century.

The Barentuma Oromo of north, northeastern, and southern Oromia and Somali regions are known as the 'Afran Qallo', 'Ittu', 'Anniyya', 'Wallo', 'Arsi', 'Karrayyu', and 'Qallu.' They are organized through a segmentary patrilineal structure of the Barentuma branch or eastern division of the great Oromo confederacy. Oromo oral history states that the confederacy was born out of the union of Xabboo and Hayo Meeto, the original Oromo father and mother, and propagated through their two sons Barentuma (Barentu) and Boran (Borana). Except for the Karrayu in the Upper and Middle Awash Rift Valley, and the Arsi in the Arsi and Bale regions, the Barentuma Oromo have largely given up pastoralism and their indigenous governance system, known as *raba-dori* or *gadaa*.[10] The *gadaa* system is a complex political and philosophical governing body traditionally based on a generational and age-grade system whereby all men born within a distinct eight-year period are of a common age set who move through a generational cycle of forty years (five age sets). While *gadaa* was outlawed during the Egyptian Occupation of Harar (1875–1885) and the rule of Abyssinian Emperor Menelik II (1887–1913), symbolic elements of the practice continue to exist today in modified form throughout Oromia.

The research for this chapter focuses mainly on the descendants of the Barentuma lineage near the city of Harar, known as the 'Afran Qallo' (literally, 'the Four Sons of Qallo'). Each *gosa* (clan) traces its line of descent to Alla, Obborra, Baabile, or Daga. Once referred to as 'Qottu' ('Those Who Dig'), the Afran Qallo are principally rural agriculturalists today. Like the derogatory term 'Galla', also used to designate 'Oromo' but not used by the Oromo themselves, the term 'Qottu' today is considered belittling and it is no longer used in contemporary scholarship (Kabir 1995, 3; Ibsa Ahmed 2011, 6). My research conducted in 2010 with other Barentuma Oromo groups (Ittu, Anniyya, Wallo, Arsi, Karrayyu) is used to explore ideas about women's dress among the Afran Qallo.

Genealogy

Barentuma (Barentu) and Boran (Borana), the sons of the great father Xabboo and the Great Mother Hayo Meeto, are considered the founding fathers of all Oromo people, and from their propagation stem numerous lineages.[11] The following is a synopsis of the Oromo genealogy (recorded in graph form in Figures 2.2 and 2.3) told by a group of elders from the Baabile *gosa*:

> The Afran Qallo trace their line of decent to Borana and Barentu, the sons of Xabboo and Meeto. Barentu was a wandering warrior while his brother, Borana, sat in one place, made peace, and begot nine sons. Barentu eventually moved east to make war. He had five sons whom he named Humbanna, Karayyu, Marawwa, Xummuga, and Akkichu. Of these, Akkichu violated Oromo law and he was banished to the eastern border of Oromia. Akkichu was very innovative. He modernized his people, invented irrigation, and had trade contacts with India through the Somali coast. But when the sons

of Barentu called him to three meetings and he failed to appear, he was excommunicated and presented with the following curse: "Just as the waters of Jijija [in your kingdom] don't flow toward the east, may the Akkichu not return to the Oromo."[12] After this, the Akkichu groups scattered far and wide. Some took oaths and joined other Oromo groups while others went east and joined the Western Somali. Some Akkichu groups went south and joined the Maasai in Kenya and the Tutsi in Rwanda (a subgroup that Oromo claim were once the Oromo *warra* 'Tuuti'). When Akkichu was ex-communicated, Barentu adopted another son called 'Qallo' in order to maintain five sons, a significant number in Oromo astronomy. Qallo had four sons with his two wives: Obborra, Daga, Alla, and Baabile. The mother of Daga, Baabile, and Obborra is named 'Kuuloo', while the mother of Alla is Karroo. These sons are known collectively as 'the four sons of Qallo' or Afran Qallo. Daga had three sons called 'Nole', 'Jarso', and 'Hume' (A.I., K.U., Q.U.H. February 14, 2000)

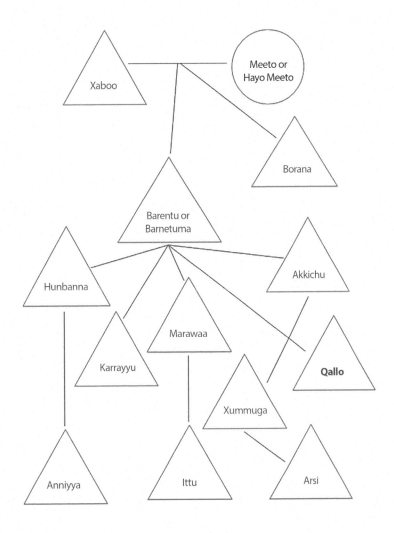

Figure 2.2 Oromo Genealogy. Figure Source: Adapted from Kabir 1995:14

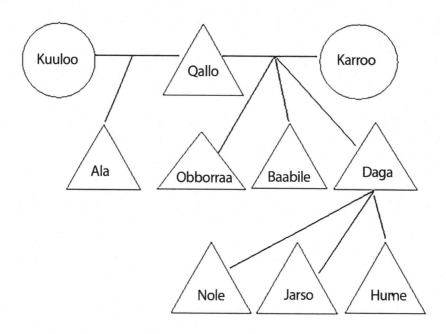

Figure 2.3 Afran Qallo Genealogy

This account makes several important points that are often brought up in discussions of genealogy. First, the great Oromo confederacy is personified through the brothers Borana (Boran) and Barentu (Barentuma) as agents of peace and war respectively. This division of responsibility is the model for the Afran Qallo's original governing assembly and generational system, *raba-dori*. *Raba* is the council of elected elders and *dori* is the military (Hassen 1973, 24). Secondly, the depiction of the son Akkichu contains within it several important points about Oromo social structure, including the centrality of adoption (*moggaasaa*) as a means to expand families, as well as political and geographic influence; the fluidity of political networks through the formation of new allegiances, including connection with other East African pastoralist groups; the severity of breaking an oath; and the banishment of perpetrators through a curse and excommunication.[13] Lastly, what is well illustrated in this passage and key for this discussion is the role that women play in this genealogical narrative. While descent is organized along a segmentary patrilineal and patrilocal stem, the names and deeds of female ancestors in Oromo history are clearly present. Leaving them out of any genealogy misses half the equation.

It is crucial for a Barentuma man to be able to recite his genealogy from memory with some skill for it will ultimately guide him in his marriage, his political alliances and estrangements, and his participation in a welfare network. In fact, it is not unusual for men to be able to remember the names of at least a dozen forefathers and a few foremothers. In traditional law, marriage is exogamous and it is only permissible between two people who are separated by blood relations by at least five generations. Subsequently, all men can remember the names and immediate relations of their great-great-grandfathers. While Oromo women marry into a *gosa* other than their own and are not required to be able to trace their blood genealogy, I found that most women could readily recite the names of between five and ten generations of ancestors, too.

In the past, the *gadaa* or *raba-dori* system served as the most central mnemonic device for remembering the past. As each *gadaa* group moved into a new grade every eight years, time was orally recorded by the Oromo name of the grade, for example Kilole *gadaa* (1538–1546), Bifole *gadaa* (1546–1554), and Michelle *gadaa* (1554–1562) (Hassen 1983, 184). Since this institution has not been practiced in most Barentuma groups for several generations, most informants that I spoke with did not use this chronological sequence. Oral histories during this early period are usually characterized through truncated accounts that center only on select meaningful events. Certainly, the distant past, particularly stories about initial contacts or first migrations, are heavily invested in present issues of citizenship and rights. Most historians would agree that an oral historical chronology that extends beyond 100 to 150 years is likely uneven in accuracy, and certainly the telescoping of past events that are no longer meaningful to the present creates a chronological bias (Henige 1974, 5). However, my concern here is not to create a historical reconstruction of the Barentuma past. Rather, I intend to relate what is collectively significant to the Oromo in their understanding of the past and how this information is visibly expressed through their body art today. Two themes emerge when Oromo elders discussed the dress of their ancestors: foreign relations and trade.

Oromo dress has been shaped by an array of imported trade goods, including textiles, ornaments, and cosmetics that come into the markets in and around Harar from India and the Middle East, and more recently from Taiwan and China. Just as imported enamelware and plastic containers are today replacing indigenous fiber baskets and black pottery, many manufactured items have taken the place of locally produced dress worn by women in the past. Yet, these imports must visually or symbolically find meaning within an Oromo identity. In interviews conducted with women, they explained that while they are faced with more and more choices in self-presentation, they have a responsibility to hold onto the visual markers that connect them to their family, clan, and ethnic group. With the influx of social, political, religious, and economic changes brought about during the Egyptian presence and the early Amhara invasion period, dress is one of the few visual remnants of the past that is called upon continually to invoke genealogical and ethnic connections.

The Oromo Migration to the Central Highland and the Early City-State of Harar

Harar had already been in existence for at least a few centuries when the Oromo arrived in the Central and Somali plateau of present-day East Hararghe zone. Harar was one of seven Muslim city-states in the Horn of Africa during the thirteenth century. As part of the Zeila confederacy dominated by the Sultanate of Ifat, Harar was an important middle point for trade caravans between the Gulf of Aden and the Ethiopian interior. After Ifat had been defeated by the Christian Kingdom of Ethiopia during the first half of the fourteenth century, the ruling delegation of Ifat, known as 'Walasma', moved the center of their power to the lowlands of Adal. It was during the fifteenth century that the capital of Adal was moved to Dakar, east of Harar and then, in 1520, Harar became the political capital of the Sultanate of Adal. By 1577, the Adal rulers had again moved their capital to the Danakil Desert, this time to avoid attacks by semi-nomadic Oromo pastoralists, and Harar became an independent city-state under the Ali ibn Daub dynasty (1647–1875) (Hassen 1980, 228).

Many history books still read by Ethiopian schoolchildren today unanimously attribute the great Oromo expansion into the Ethiopian Plateau and the Central Highlands, and specifically the movement of the Afran Qallo Oromo into the Juba and Webe Shebelli River Valleys, to a mass exodus in the sixteenth century from outside present-day Ethiopia; a moment in time when warring Muslim and Christian factions were exhausted. It is more likely that the Afran Qallo Oromo gradually resettled in this region over time from southern Ethiopia (Hassen 2017, 123). This is particularly credible since no corroborating oral confirmations exist, and since there is no evidence of any kind of technological or agricultural advances that would have spurred a tidal wave of movement (Melbaa 1988, 6). By the early 1570s, it is clear that the Afran Qallo had moved with some permanence to just beyond the Harari gardens outside the city wall of Harar. A written source gathered by an Italian governor in Harar, Enrico Cerulli (1936, 36), indicates that the Harari emir Nur ibn Mujahid, encountered Oromo soldiers in 1559 in Harar when he returned from a battle with Christian highlanders in Abyssinia. Emir Nur is subsequently credited with the construction of a wall to deter Oromo forces who "in the next eight years . . . had reduced the political and trading domain of the "Adal capital of Harar to such an extent that only the city itself survived" (Waldron 1984, 23).[14]

Relations between the Oromo and the Harari during this early contact period in the Emirate of Harar were riddled with strife (Yusuf Ahmed 1960; Abbas Ahmed 1992; Caulk 1977; Hassen 1973, 1999). By the nineteenth century, Harari soldiers were constantly raiding the Oromo populations beyond the wall in order to collect taxes and safeguard Harari-owned gardens and caravan routes, while Oromo forces continued to try to stabilize their communities near Harar and gain a foothold in the local economy. An example of the hostilities between the groups is illustrated in a song that dates to the reign of Emir Ahmed ibn Abu Bakr (1756–1783), who unsuccessfully tried to subdue the Oromo (called 'Galla' at the time of his rule). The Harari song states: "Ululate to him, insert a feather on his head, your father's son has killed a Galla" (Gadid 1979, 29). A feather added to the hair was a way to show bravery at the taking of a life; perhaps a symbol that may have been adopted either from the Oromo, the Somali or the Afar, who traditionally wore "feathers in their hair after killing" (Hassen 2017, 89–90).

Muslim campaigns into the Oromo territories were already being organized and taking root, particularly under the proselytizing zeal of the successor Emir Abd-al

Shakur (1783–1794), who introduced currency and administrative reforms. This drew the Oromo into tighter dependence on the emirate. Emir Abdulkarim (1825–1834) encouraged fuller participation of the Oromo in the commercial culture of the city through their production of saffron, coffee, and wheat (Garad 1979, 49). At the time of British explorer Richard Burton's visit in 1854, Emir Abu Bakr (1852–1856) allowed the Nole and other Oromo farmers to sell coffee, *khat*, tobacco, and safflower in the city markets but taxed them on their land and harvests to such an extent that Oromo women were forced to travel weekly to the markets to sell their produce for the needed currency with which to pay the tariffs. Emir Muhammed (1856–1875), himself from an Oromo family, brought Oromo into tighter commercial trading relations with the Harari through the planting of new cash crops, the building of mosques, and the introduction of Muslim missionaries into Oromo communities (Hassen 1999, 21, 25–27). Through the indigenous institution of the adoption of foreigners into Oromo clans, Muslim missionaries began to serve as mediators in local disputes.

Concerning the early historical accounts mentioned above, Oromo oral tradition is vague. When asked when the Oromo first arrived in Harar, for example, informants' usual answer placed the Afran Qallo arrival in Harar at the time of the Arab Shaykh Abadir al-Rida, who is renowned by the Harari, Argobba, and Oromo as the patron saint of Harar. He is believed to have traveled to Harar from Arabia around the mid-tenth century (Gibb 1996: 81).[15] Shaykh Abadir is remembered for his Islamic proselytizing, and for consolidating the ethnically diverse communities around Harar through Islamic conversion. A group of Nole elders recounted how Shaykh Abadir gave the Nole and Ala Oromo the first string of wooden prayer beads, the Arabic called *tasbii* (M.S.S. February 27, 2002).

This account of the Nole alliance with Shaykh Abadir and his gift to them of *tasbii* (prayer beads) aligns the Oromo with the early Islamic, urban complex of Harar and the coalescence of various groups under the control of an illustrious ruler. The wearing and fingering of a strand of wooden beads during prayer may even function as a tactile remembrance of the historical placing of the Oromo and Harari side by side during the time of Abadir under the roof of Islam. For most Oromo with whom I spoke, the memories of past events, whether migration, war, or religious conversion, are not defined by calendrical dates, but rather are linked to the lifespan of notable people and their heroic deeds, and articulated through personal objects. The names of heroes, ancestors, and spiritual advisors through which events of the past are understood and remembered are also visually realized in dress.

The *Sabbata* and the Great Oromo Mother, Hayo Meeto

It is this distant past of the Oromo migration into the Central Highlands that is recalled in the tying of the *sabbata* (a woman's belt) at the waist. Throughout many regions of Oromia, the belt is given to a young woman at marriage by her mother or an older woman who has not been divorced. While this wrapping is herein discussed in connection with the Afran Qallo, the women's belt plays a central role for all Barentuma Oromo women, in addition to serving as a sign of marriage and fecundity, to indicate the historical positioning of these Afran Qallo Oromo on the landscape and their proprietorial claims to those land and resources.

Today, the voluminous folds of all women's dresses in Oromia are held in place by the *sabbata*. When wearing this traditional dress of *saddetta* (white sheeting) the tying of *sabbata* at the waist requires three key steps. First, the cloth of the *saddetta* is fitted over the *sabbata*. Once on the body, the outer folds of the *saddetta* are lifted and tied at the shoulder to cover the torso. At marriage, the length of the *sabbata* is ritually wrapped around the waist repeatedly, dependent on the waist size, while reiterating claims of the ancestors and then tied together. The remaining ties hang loosely down at the front of the abdomen and the material is bloused over the *sabbata*. Since the folds of the *saddetta* drape over the sash, either the *sabbata* will be totally invisible or only the ends of the sash will be slightly exposed. Owing to its placement under the sagging weight of a Barentuma woman's dress, the *sabbata* is often partially or completely concealed. Since the modern sash is neither locally woven nor often visible today, I regarded it upon first examination as merely a trifle bit of cloth necessary to hold women's dresses in place. The silky texture of the contemporary Afran Qallo sash and the names of its specific types, the darker *manqux* worn by young women and the whiter *durriya* worn by older women, suggested to me the potential for profitable information on the Red Sea trade with Harar. However, informants continually brushed off my questions about where the imported *sabbata* originated with a dismissive "from outside."

While I encountered a variety of belt styles often made with imported materials throughout north, east and central Oromia, Barentuma women insisted that their belts were a central part of a woman's traditional dress. Among the Afran Qallo, the sash was originally woven locally. Today's *sabbata* is made from imported, strip-woven cloth approximately twelve inches wide and three to five-and-a-half yards long (Figure 2.4). Those fashionable among other Barentuma women today can range in type from machine-made plastic in Wallo to loom-woven cloth with multi-colored tassels among the Ittu. One Karrayyu woman at the weekly market scolded me for not photographing her white, plastic belt, explaining its importance with the words: "We are modern, like our mothers."

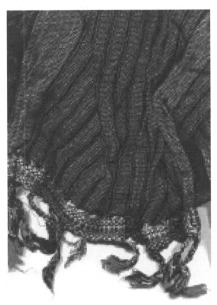

Figure 2.4 An Oromo Woman's Sabbata

The reference to mothers is also symbolically expressed in the actions of belting or tying the cloth around the waist. Hayo Meeto, the mother of Barentu and Borana, and her role in the Barentuma migration are embodied in this belt that binds the belly, as well as the use of *sabbata* as a metaphor for migration and consolidating. Oromo oral tradition states that it was the responsibility of the Great Mother Hayo Meeto to divide the land for her five grandchildren, the sons of Barentu. As tradition states, she sat down in Hirna, a town west of Harar, which would become the central meeting place for the five sons of Barentu. There, Hayo Meeto began to wind a *sabbata* around her waist five times. She encouraged the young women from the area to take a piece of long cloth and follow suit. As she encircled her waist, Hayo Meeto prophesied the regional distribution of land for her grandsons with each wrap of the cloth:

> Hunbanna should have the land near Qunbii
> Murawwa should have the region from Gawgaw to Ancaar
> Xummuga should have Did'aa and Baale
> Karayyu should have the area of Hadaama and Harsadee
> Qallo should have the land from Chercher to Balal.[16]

The young women are said to have watched attentively and followed her motions. When Hayo Meeto finished speaking and wrapping, the girls took her to her home in Walaabu[17] and sang: "The places chosen by the mother are now clear."[18] This line is still repeated during certain wedding songs sung by old women to the mother of the bride the night before the marriage ceremony.

Qallo's son's land was further divided by three female leaders from Walaabu: Rooboo Halloo, Shaadiraa Boruu, and Maroo Jiloo. Whether these women were the wives of Qallo was not something my research collaborators could verify; they were only described as great ancestors whose names had been preserved. These women continued the tradition of Hayo Meeto and divided the land through song as they wrapped their *sabbata*. This time they encircled their waists four times and sang:

> Daga should have Wareeris
> Baabile should have Mullu
> Obborra should have Obbi
> Alla should have Mullata.[19]

The stories of Hayo Meeto, the Great Mother, and the female elders at Walaabu reflect the symbolic importance of the wrapping of the waist as a metaphor for the claiming and legitimizing of the Afran Qallo homeland, described today as the fertile "belly" of the valley west of Harar. The final tie of the *sabbata* symbolically seals the aforementioned locations for the Qallo patrilineage. When Afran Qallo women dress in *saddetta*, they repeat the actions of the Great Mother and other female ancestors before them, consciously re-enacting the migration narrative (Figures 2.5). Today, the *sabbata* is not usually long enough to encircle the waist more than twice. Only one kind of *sabbata*, called 'sabbata mudhi,' is intended to be wrapped around the waist four or five times. Albeit in modified form, the wrapping itself is a daily reminder of the division of land granted the Afran Qallo descendants. While the egalitarian nature of the *raba-dori* assembly allowed women in the past to participate in political decision making and play a modified role in the generational system with men, today they are restricted by the court of Shari'a (the fundamental religious concept of Islam, namely its law) and the Ethiopian government in these processes. The personal roping of the sash connects them back to the political power of the Great Mother. In this sense, the symbolic action of tying also recognizes an Afran Qallo woman's historic ability to pass laws, contain mandates, and maintain these rules.

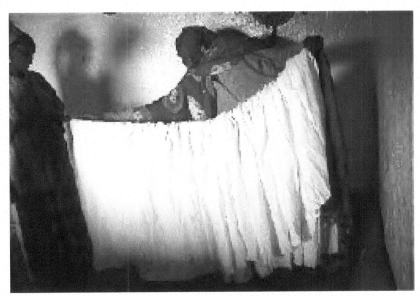

Figure 2.5 Placing the Cloth Saddetta onto the Belt Sabbata

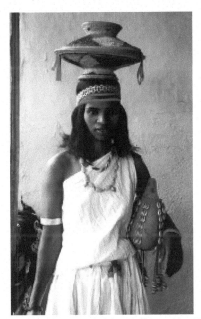

Figure 2.6 The Cloth Saddetta bloused over the Belt Sabbata

The tying of the *sabbata* is also seen as a way of acknowledging and protecting the potency of the belly. By securing the mid-section, the area associated with the ideals of girth and fecundity, is both harnessed and emphasized. In Oromo thought, this is an important locus of power from where the Afran Qallo lineage is preserved. Yet, it is largely concealed under the dress it binds. The wrapping and tying of the *sabbata* by young women are therefore also a means of keeping safe the region ripe with the potential to bear a descendant. Lastly, this region also connects a woman to Waqaa, the almighty, traditional celestial deity. The Oromo call the rainbow 'sabbata Waqaajo' (literally, 'the binding of God's stomach'). As a woman wraps sabbata around her life-giving belly, the rainbow binds the heavenly midsection of God.[20]

The sabbata is an item of dress that has morphed materially from leather to locally produced cotton to foreign manufacture. In this sense, it is also iconic of the changes taking place in the historical period in and around Harar.

Richard Burton, Philip Paulitschke, and the Mercantile Landscape of Harar

When foreign travelers first negotiated the terrain of present-day eastern Ethiopia, they came across an assortment of costumes among the people they visited, including the soft leather uwa or wadaroo, finely woven cotton tobes (Arabic for 'cloth'), ornate filigree silver ornaments, and plaited hairstyles prepared with clarified butter. Wherever they went, foreign cloth was in high demand. We know from early travelers' accounts that the Muslim states of southwestern Ethiopia were involved in the cloth trade that came from the coast through Harar, and returned with slaves, mules and horses from at least the time of Portuguese contact in the fifteenth century. Exotic textiles from India, Arabia, Europe, and Turkey also made their way into the royal and elite costumes in the Christian kingdoms of the Abyssinian Kingdom (Pankhurst 1961, 255).

Two explorers took the liberty to record in great detail the fashions they encountered among the Oromo: the British explorer Sir Richard Burton, who reached Harar in 1854; and the Austrian ethnographer Dr. Philip Paulitschke, who traveled throughout what is present-day Oromia in the mid-1880s. They have left behind several descriptions, sketches, and photographs that illuminate aspects of regional dress, including trade, aesthetic sensibility, stylistic choices, and technologies, such as metallurgy and weaving, that are useful for this study. Richard Burton's accounts of trade items and descriptions of dress serve as an excellent starting point to reconstruct dress in the Horn of Africa prior to the mid-nineteenth century. However, before addressing his writings on the Oromo, I want to share the dress that he himself wore. Burton was a keen observer of appearances, as noted in his writings, and his own clothing choices were integral to his survival in a rather inhospitable place for a white, Christian foreigner.

Burton was intimately aware of the politics at play between identity and costume when he pondered whether to don Muslim or European dress for his reception by the Emir of Harar in 1854. Contrary to popular opinion, he chose the garb of an Englishman instead of the Muslim attire he had worn throughout his trip. While he assured the concerned East India Company in Aden that he would travel to Harar in Muslim disguise before he departed, when he neared Harar, he changed his mind. He writes: "As I approached the city men turned out of their villages to ask if that was the Turk who was going to his death? The question made me resolve to appear before the Emir in my own character, an Englishman . . . as a rule, the Ottoman is more hated and feared than the Frank. On the 3rd of January I entered Harar" (Burton

1855, 143). Burton understood that a turban and Arabic dress might incite the Emir. Furthermore, he knew from experience that the local demand for the raw materials he carried, such as indigo-dyed cloth, coarse canvas, calico, and white beads, were the foundations of costumes of particular clans and, as such, an arrangement of these materials would clearly state one's origins to neighboring groups. He writes that "all the races amongst whom my travels lay, hold him nidering [dastardly] who hides his origin in places of danger; and secondly, my white face had converted me into a Turk, a nation more hated and suspected than any European" (Burton 1987, 197). Therefore, he changed his clothes. We learn that people were clearly interested in categorizing Burton through his clothes and complexion at each new place to which he ventured:

> This fairness, and the Arab dress, made me at different times the ruler of Aden, the chief of Zayla, the Hajji's son, a boy, an old woman, a man painted white, a warrior in silver armour, a merchant, a pilgrim, a hedgepriest, Ahmad the Indian, a Turk, an Egyptian, a Frenchman, a Banyan, a shariff, and lastly a Calamity sent down from heaven to weary out the lives of the Somal: every kraal had some conjuncture of its own, and each fresh theory was received by my companions with roars of laughter. (Burton 1987, 120)

Burton advised travelers to Harar to know the specific kinds of materials that went into cultural costmes. He warned: "Before entering a district the traveler should ascertain what may be the especial variety [of beads]. Some kinds are greedily sought for in one place, and in another rejected with disdain" (61). In these early writings, Burton reveals not only the trade goods that were in demand in the various regions near Harar, but in his descriptions of women's costumes, he emphasizes the significant regional and cultural preferences placed on art of the body by the Oromo, Somali, and Harari peoples he encountered.

We learn from Paulitschke (1888b, 261) thirty years later that Oromo women's fashions, particularly their leather dress and hairstyle, were so distinct from neighboring dress, that in the late nineteenth century, Harari and Arab slave traders used it to their advantage to disguise their slaves as Oromo peasants. Since the Oromo in and around Harar did not practice slavery and were not involved in the trade, by dressing slaves as Oromo, slave caravans would not be regarded with suspicion, especially during the Egyptian Occupation when slavery was firmly outlawed but still surreptitiously practiced (Paulitschke 1888b, 261).[21] The slave trade that ran from the Ethiopian interior to the coast was an important part of Harar's economy during the nineteenth century; for example, Gurage girls from the Abyssinian interior fetched the highest price in the slave markets – eighty thalers. Boys between the ages of nine and ten years were sold for thirty to thirty-five thalers (Paulitschke 1888b: 262). When smuggling slaves from the interior to Harar and from Harar to Zeila and Berbera, slavers dressed their female captives in the leather clothes of Oromo women and dressed their male slaves in the hand-woven tunics worn by Oromo men (Paulitschke 1888b, 261). Specifically, female captives were made to wear *uwa*, the classic Oromo leather dress consisting of a softened hide belted at the waist and secured at the shoulder. While the dress is eventually transformed into a cotton wrapper (1875–1885) by decree from the Egyptian colonial administration, the *uwa* and the leather waist tie remain the prototype for the cloth ensembles of today, worn in the latest fashionable rayon and polyester prints in and near the city of Harar.

On his approach on horseback to Harar in 1854, Richard Burton, who was supported by the East India Company to conduct an expedition from Berbera to Harar, advanced through several Oromo farming communities at the fringes of the great wall. He observed: "[U]p to the city gates the country is peopled by [Oromo]. This unruly race requires to be propitiated by presents of cloth; as many as 600 Tobes are annually distributed amongst them by the Emir" (Burton 1987, 19 vol. II). A *tobe* is a man's cloth, worn wrapped around the torso in the fashion of a Roman toga. As early as the 1780s, the Harari Emir, Abd-al Shakur (1783–1794), gathered locally woven cloth and "went with a friend to the Jarso and other Nole clans . . . in order to civilize them." (Caulk 1977, 372)

While Jarso and Nole men may have been wearing leather garments like their women during the time of Emir Abd-al Shakur, one hundred years later, Oromo men were weaving and wearing a cotton cloth, some nine yards long by two yards wide.

We know from early explorers and administrators that a successful weaving industry existed in Harar. Harari male weavers produced high-quality white and red cotton cloth, and sashes from at least the late eighteenth century onward. Burton (1987, 27–28) writes:

> The Tobes and sashes of Harar are considered equal to the celebrated cloth of Shoa: hand-woven, they as far surpass, in beauty and durability, the vapid produce of European manufactories, as the perfect hand of man excels the finest machine. On the windward coast, one of these garments is considered a handsome present for a chief . . . They are made of the fine, long-stapled cotton, which grows plentifully upon these hills, and are soft as silk, whilst their warmth admirably adapts them for winter wear. The thread is spun by women with two wooden pins; the loom is worked by both sexes.

In the 1880s Paulitschke (1896, 52) found that the finest cloth for men's *chuchu* (*tobe*) was produced by Oromo weavers from the finest Oromo-grown cotton and fetched a high price. The exact price is not mentioned, but he does tell us that a *chuchu*[22] of imported cloth and poor quality cost only one Maria Theresa thaler in Harar, while an Oromo weaver was given an entire cow as payment for a *tobe* measuring five yards in length (52). He writes: [F]for the Afar and Somali, the [Oromo] weaves are regarded as real treasures and they are sold in Shoa, Abyssinia, Harar, and also on the northern and eastern Somali coast for a good price" (80).

The Egyptians initially found male Oromo weavers outside of Harar weaving fine cloth on a *qeeba* (a wooden pit-treadle loom) (Figure 2.7). Their wives and daughters gathered the cotton from Harari landowners on plots outside the city, and cleaned the seeds from the cotton with a wooden instrument known as a '*bu'aa*' and spun the cotton on a spool called '*indirtii*' made from pieces of wood and calabash (A.A.J. April 4, 2000). Yet, by the end of the Egyptian Occupation in 1885, the Oromo relied almost entirely on the town's imported textiles, and loom weaving fell into disuse.[23] All weaving in Harar came to a halt by the late nineteenth century (Pankhurst 1964, 224). In the 1880s, cloth from India and the United Sates was brought in large bales to the market, and then cut into men's *tobe*s. One *tobe* measured nine yards long and two yards wide, and usually cost one Maria Theresa thaler (Paulitschke 1888b, 260). However, the cloth from Yemen was more expensive, costing from twenty to twenty-five thalers for a bale of sixty-six yards (260).[24] Despite the saturation of cloth from America, India, and Arabia, locally produced cloth was of much higher quality and preferred by the Oromo, Harari, and Somali populations throughout the second half of the nineteenth century. These groups were also willing to pay a higher price for it (261). Paulitschke (1896, 80) presented several textiles from Harar to the natural history museum in Vienna upon his return to Austria in the late 1880s that "were looked at by experts and pegged the best cotton weaving that exists in the excellent fiber, thread, and craftsmanship."[25]

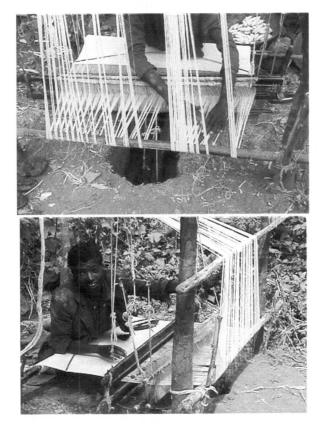

Figure 2.7 A Pit-Treadle Loom

Despite the preference for locally produced, high-quality cloth, Nole Oromo elders recounted how the Harari rulers actually outlawed the Oromo-made white cloth with a red border, locally known in Harari as *ifat iras*, that was made by, and for, men so that the Oromo would purchase imported materials (I.A. February 20, 2000). Others mentioned that during the Egyptian Occupation, only very elderly men, who could not afford the imported cloth and who knew the weaving process, continued to make cloth on their looms (M.W.G. February 1, 2000). Owing, in part, to the increasing presence of cheap, manufactured textiles in Harar, and the regulations imposed by the government requiring locals to stop manufacturing their own cloth and to adopt it, the Oromo weaving industry was in a rapid state of decline by the later part of the nineteenth century. Today, the cloth cottage industry has been completely taken over by male Harari and Gurage tailors who line the path from Feres Magala to Magala Gudo in Harar, and sew clothes from imported cloth. Singer sewing machines were bought by Harari merchants as early as 1909 (Pankhurst 1964, 226). The last Oromo woven cloth and knowledge of weaving in the Harar region are things of the past.

During Burton's time, perhaps because of the overabundance of currency, specific kinds of cloth (*wolati, merikani, hindi*) and locally made *tobe*s were used as the principal trade medium for produce, animals, and wares. In the 1850s, Burton (1987, 170) reports that "the price of a good camel varies from six to eight clothes; one Tobe buys a two-year-old heifer, three, a cow between three and four years old. A ewe costs half a cloth." As is true of much of the imported materials in Harar, these trade clothes were often named after the place from which they originated: Bombei (Geganafi): Harari women's embroidered trousers with threads from India; Merikati: American sheeting; Kutch: cotton from the West Indian state; Calicut or Calico: patterned, plain-woven cotton cloth from Calcutta; Gujarati: cloth from Gujarat in Northwest India; Jiddawi: black cloth from Jiddah; Shinabii: silk dress from China; and Buckram: a stiff coarse cotton from Bukhara in southwest Asia. Along with the merchant economy of Harar that brought the names of foreign places, the tongue of the Arabic travelers also affixed itself to local dress: *tasbii* (wooden prayer beads), *foota* (dress), *qarxasaa* (leather talisman), and *henna* (plant dye). The names of adornment attest to both the long distance the items had to travel and their Arabic origins, granting the owner cosmopolitan and Muslim prestige.

Even as Oromo women living near Harar were trading in the great variety of cloth types mentioned above, they did not yet wear them themselves. As one official in the Egyptian government in Harar reported, Oromo men living on the outskirts of the city were dressed in cloth, while Oromo women wore only leather costumes (Moktar 1876, 383). In his descriptions of women's dress in the countryside among the Gudabirsi Somali and Oromo in 1854, Burton (1987, 137) finds women outfitted in "a petticoat of hides [which] made no great mystery of forms." Yet, as the following section demonstrates, women participated in the cottage industry of textile production in Harar through the harvesting of cotton, and the spinning and weaving of textiles until its decline in the 1880s. Despite their closeness to the production of textiles, the trade in cloth, and the wearing of cloth *tobe*s by their fathers, sons, husbands, and female neighbors, the transformation of their leather *uwa* to the cloth *saddetta* was slow in coming, while it appears that neighboring

Somali women ivory traders had already cast aside their leather clothes for *merikani* fabrics decades earlier (Akou 2011, 33). Why is it that these Oromo women, who certainly had cloth at their disposal, did not begin to adopt the wearing of textiles until sometime between the 1890s and the 1920s? What prompted this transition from animal skin to cloth around the turn of the century? What are the historical links between leather garments and the manufactured dresses worn today?

The Transition from Leather to Cloth in Oromo Women's Dress: The Egyptian Occupation of Harar (1875–1885)

Twenty years after Burton's departure from Harar, Egyptian forces invaded the walled city. The Egyptians were initially interested in the city-state of Harar because of its prominence as a trading center, its geographical location along several East African trade routes, and its opening onto the Ethiopian interior, a point from which the Nile River could be secured (Paulitschke 1888b, 237). Their ten-year occupation had a profound effect on Oromo dress: the abrupt shift by Oromo men from the wearing of locally woven cloth to the exclusive use of imported materials, and the transformation of women's garments from leather to cloth.

When Ismail Pasha, the leader of Egypt from 1863 to 1879, decided to tighten his control in the Red Sea and, by extension, Ethiopia, he began by capturing the Red Sea ports of Masawwa, Berbera and Zeila. In October 1875, the Egyptian troops reached Gurgura, where the Nole Oromo unsuccessfully fought them in a seven-hour battle. After almost three hundred years of independence, Harar came under Egyptian rule as Emir Mohammed surrendered peacefully when Ismail Pasha's army arrived at the city gates. The chiefs of the Oromo bands who had tried unsuccessfully to push the foreigners back at the outskirts of the city were immediately imprisoned and forced to "dissolve their parliament, deliver up their Abba Bokku, cut off their *dufura*s or long hair, and submit to circumcision. A great number preferred to be killed rather than be thus humiliated, but after three or four years they were reduced to such misery that the majority submitted. That was the end of Oromo supremacy in south-eastern Ethiopia" (Trimingham 1965, 121).

During the Egyptian period, rural peoples were first subject to the effects of severe taxation, massive Islamic conversion, land reform, and new material goods (Hassen 1980, 224). One fifth of the one million Oromo inhabitants who lived just beyond the walls of Harar at the time were forced into paying taxes to the Khedive (Moktar cited in Caulk 1977, 371). The Egyptians imposed a tax called '*zaka*' on all domestic animals and goods. For every pack animal, a fee of five piasters (the new Egyptian currency) was required, and to bring in or take out wares such as hides, a toll was paid in each direction (Paulitschke 1888b, 251). Although the Oromo "head tax" to enter the city, called the '*Galla mahaleq*' after the local Harari coin, had been abolished, many Oromo lost their land due to the high *zaka* tax (238, 251).

The coastal caravans containing trade goods coming to Harar also increased six-fold, from seventy caravans annually during the time of the emirs to four hundred under the Egyptians due to the establishment of way stations and improved defense, and any new items of dress inundated the Harar markets (Paulitschke 1887, 588). At the same time, as caravans from the east began pouring into Harar, several merchants from Turkey, Syria, Yemen, and India came to Harar to set up shop, particularly bakeries and leather kiosks (588). These individuals also provided visual models of new costume types. While the Oromo recall the plethora of new dress styles available during the time of their grandparents and great-grandparents and their special fascination with the dress of the Egyptian soldiers, they say that as tax-paying subjects, their ancestors needed to visually fit into the Oromo tax-paying class. Since many Oromo men at this time shared a common dress style with their Harari and Somali neighbors, it appears that the Egyptians were thinking particularly of the women's *saddetta* as an organizing principle for Oromo recognition and quick tax collecting.[26] Women state that Egyptian administrators came with an official decree to Oromo villages some ten to fifteen miles from Harar, demanding that Oromo women wear cloth wrappers or be fined. Women remember stories handed down from their great-grandmothers in which Oromo women, who heard the news of the decree, ran to find any spare pieces of cloth with which to cover their torsos before the officials arrived (M.M. March 10, 2000; J.A. February 3, 2000). Like European colonial administrations in other parts of Africa, the Egyptian rulers also regarded their presence in Harar as a civilizing mission, and enforced cloth not only to regulate the diverse populations and bind them more tightly into the commerce of Harar, but also to spread Qur'anic ideas of morality, modesty, and the covering of the body.

According to women informants, the Egyptians only allowed Muslim women into Harar to buy and sell in the markets. Those women who approached the city wearing tanned hides were turned away at the gate and criticized for not accepting Islam (N.A.M. March 18, 2000). While most women did not yet abandon their leather *uwa* entirely, they did begin wrapping imported sheeting around their upper bodies, which they secured with leather straps for quick costume changes that would allow them to attend the market (J.A. February 3, 2000).

The Egyptian period saw intensive brutality and bloodshed against the Oromo: a pyramid of Oromo skulls in front of the gates to the city bore testimony to the Egyptian ruler's severity. Rauf Pasha, the first governor of the city, recruited Somali forces to attack Oromo opposition forces, kill them, and return with their heads. Many Oromo recounted the names of leaders they lost, including Caamaa Nuur, the leader of Jarso and Huumee; Ballaa Buuba, the leader of the Nole; and Waday Kormoosoo, the leader of the Alla, the Oromo. They were also forced to stop going to the sacred grounds at Walaabu for the meetings of their general *raba-dori* assembly where laws were established, court cases heard, and connections to other Oromo groups renewed. The bridge between the Barentuma Oromo pastoralists who were beyond the control of the Egyptian state and the Afran Qallo Oromo agriculturalists near the city intensified.

The Afran Qallo made another unsuccessful attempt to topple the Egyptian government in 1878 under the reign of Nadi Pasha, the second governor of Harar. A force of no fewer than 35,000 Oromo surrounded the city walls in an attempt to starve the enemy into surrender, but they were defeated by a contingent of Egyptian soldiers arriving from the coast (Paulitschke 1888b, 232). The soldiers also took prisoner the president of the *raba-dori* assembly, who was later converted to Islam and used as an instrument of Egyptian assimilation policies (Hassen 1973, 23).

The disintegration of the indigenous governing system, one founded on democratic principles and organized around a largely pastoral livelihood, created for the Oromo a severe rupture with the past. It is said that at this time the story of the primordial mother Hayo Meeto and the cloth *sabbata* was born. Afran Qallo women had themselves just begun to replace their leather belts with loom-woven cloth sashes. By associating this new material with Hayo Meeto, who wrapped cloth around her waist to distribute land to her sons, Afran Qallo women were reclaiming this new dress code as their own. Similarly, women's forced adoption of a cloth garment to identify them as Muslim, to be allowed to trade, and to pay taxes during the Egyptian Occupation was also visually transformed into a meaningful symbol. The defunct practices of the traditional religion and government, *raba-dori*, and pastoralism were reified as nostalgic ideals in the cloth dress of women through their visual connection to the leather garments that "all Oromo women wore when they were free" (K.A.M. March 12, 2000).

Saddetta: The Afran Qallo Dress

The materials of an Oromo women's costume changed from leather to imported coarse canvas and then, today, to Ethiopian-produced factory cloth. The original leather skirt recorded by Burton in the 1850s became a leather skirt with a canvas wrapper in some regions by the time of Paulitschke's visits in the 1880s. Finally, by the turn of the century, a single cotton sheet became the dominant dress style among the agricultural communities with the closest contact to Harar. Yet, owing to the complex folding and tucking, all the *saddetta* styles, with their visual suggestion of two separate pieces of cloth, still contain references to the two-piece ensemble of the leather dress. Moreover, the final tie on the right shoulder visually recalls the leather strap that once held the leather skirt in place.

Oromo elders confirm that during the 1850s, all Afran Qallo women wore leather garments, a style of dress that only ceased being worn among rural female elders in Fedis and Jarso some eighty years ago (M.A.H. March 4, 2000). Paulitschke (1888b, 52), in the 1880s, describes the dress in more detail: "The women wear only a faded goatskin skirt (*uwa*) that reaches a little below the knee and under the uncovered breast. It is pulled taut and around the hips this creates a fold. The girls wear the breast covered with a leather strap over the right shoulder to secure the dress."

The historical *uwa* is a leather skirt of tanned goat, antelope or cow hide that hung to the mid-calf. The leather was rubbed with the pounded root of the Sarkama tree to dye it a deep red, and animal fat or butter was used to soften it. The hide wrapped around the waist and was secured with a leather belt, fringed at the bottom and decorated with cowry shells. The upper body was left bare in the case of older, married women but young women often wore the draped pieces of leather above the breast and secured it with a leather strap at the right shoulder, which kept the skirt in place and allowed women to transport materials and children.

Leather garments were made collectively by men and women. Men killed and skinned the animal and tanned the hide while women softened the cloth with fat, and cut and sewed the leather. Time was spent making the garment soft and well tailored. Leather anklets called '*fanta*' were also added to decorate the legs. Leather straps used to harness goods called '*naqaan qatto*' either attached to the *uwa* or criss-crossed in the front or back, and were an important part of a working woman's ensemble even after cotton dresses were worn.

As mentioned above, Oromo men readily adopted cloth to their wardrobe while women continued to dress in the animal skins that men and women had worn in the past (Hassen 1983, 198; Mohktar 1876, 383). As none of the sixteenth-century Christian and Muslim sources mention that Oromo men wore animal skins, it is likely that men may have adopted cotton cloth even before the pastoral migration in the fifteenth or sixteenth century. For instance, in the peace treaty between Emir Uthman (1567–1569) and the Oromo, it is stated clearly that the Oromo were allowed to come to the Muslim market centers and buy "cotton cloth as a fixed price" (Cerulli 1931, 58). Mohammed Hassen (1983, 198) writes: "Although it is impossible to establish with certainty just when the Oromo started to change their traditional skin clothing in favour of cotton cloth, this information [Uthman's decree] shows that cotton cloth was popular among the Oromo at the time. What can be said with certainty is that this demand for cotton cloth covered only men and not women." It is likely that Oromo communities were not only using cotton clothes, but they knew its market value and protested against its inflated prices in the market centers.

Somewhere between the Egyptian Occupation of Harar (1875–1885) and 1920, the leather skirt and the leather shoulder tie were replaced with cotton (heavy, canvas cloth) made by all Afran Qallo Oromo women. While there are pockets of Boraana Oromo in the Bale Province, where women continue to wear hide dresses and Wood (1999, 40) reports that the wearing of animal skins was prevalent as late as the 1950s among the Gabra Oromo in Northern Kenya, we no longer find Barentuma women using leather as everyday wear. Afran Qallo women's nineteenth-century *uwa* or *wadaroo* (leather dress), as described by Burton, Paulitschke, and Oromo elders, is similar in appearance to the leather garments worn today on special occasions by the Arsi, Anniyya, Ittu, and Karrayu Oromo pastoralist neighbors. The Arsi, situated between the Christian Empire and the Harari Emirate, have maintained many of the pastoralist traditions that the Afran Qallo no longer practice. I did find some women who still owned leather dresses and capes, but most of them created the look of the original leather fringed garments with brown fabric made of cotton, suede or polyester and accented with plastic beads.

When Afran Qallo women originally accepted cloth, they wore textiles only at the torso, keeping their leather *uwa*. This grouping of leather and textile is not unique to the Afran Qallo. It has also been observed among the Arsi and the western Oromo who wear leather dresses or skirts with a torso cloth even in the modern period. Pankhurst (1961, 256) reports that earlier, at the time of Almeida's visit in the late sixteenth century, poor women wore cloth and leather in Gojam and Dambea. "It was customary also for the women to wrap themselves in a 'piece of cloth' (*shamma*), though those who could not afford both wore one or other, the poorest using only dressed ox skins or even skins with the hair on, which were merely tanned till they were soft" (256). This pairing of leather with textiles, however, is unique within Ethiopia and the African Horn. In his observation of this dress, Paulitschke (1896, 79) writes: "There is present a combination of leather and cotton dress seldom found in East Africa." In one of only a few examples of this transitional dress style, an 1890s illustration shows two women working in a compound who wear the leather *uwa* but who have adopted a cloth torso wrap that leaves their shoulders exposed (Figure 2.8). This cotton torso cloth was imported from either India or North America through Zeila and was secured with the leather strap of the *uwa* on the right shoulder. The cloth bunched around the waist, creating a series of folds reminiscent of the way in which *uwa* was worn. One informant recounted that imported cotton textiles were brought by a suitor to her grandmother when her grandmother was a young girl, likely in the 1920s. She held the torso cloth in place with a leather strap (J.A. February 3, 2000).

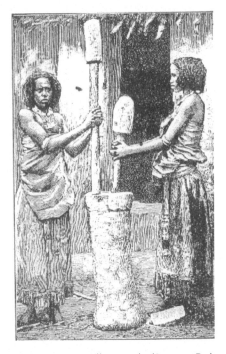

Figure 2.8 Drawing of Two Women pounding Grain (Source: Robecchi- Bricchetti 1896, 221)

A young girl situated between two boys dons this two-piece ensemble that was adopted first by young girls and later by their mothers (Figure 2.9). The skirt is tied with *sabbata* and the torso cloth is wrapped around from the back to the front and secured with a tuck between the breasts. This new dress was made of two yards or eight *waara* of cloth for the torso and two yards for the skirt. In time, the two-cloth ensemble was replaced with the single white cotton cloth four-and-a-half yards long known as '*saddetta*' (the Oromo word for the number eight as each cloth was eight *waara*). Today, the cloth is measured in *waara* (half a yard) of *lamii* (two yards), *sadii* (three yards), *afrii* (four-and-a-half yards), *shenii* (five-and-a-half yards), *saddett* (nine yards), and the dress is called by its length. A young girl, for example, would wear *afrii*.

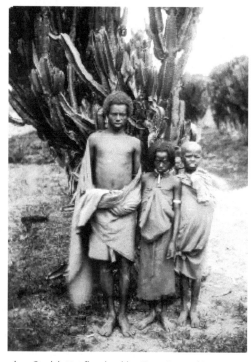

Figure 2.9 A Girl wearing Saddetta flanked by Two Boys (Source: Paulitschke 1888a, 30)

During this transition, the *saddetta* was worn at least three different ways. A photograph taken in the 1880s shows the strapless style in which four women in front of a homestead each wear a single piece of cloth wrapped around the body and gathered at the front, allowing the front of the cloth to hang loosely over the belted waist (Figure 2.10). This style mimics the two-piece ensemble. The second variant called *guddo* can be seen in a photograph by Paulitschke of roughly the same period (Figure 2.11). Here, each young woman wears a single, white cotton cloth wrapped first around her waist then over her right shoulder and finally across her torso, tucked in at the breast. The last style is the one most commonly found today among communities located near Harar (Figure 2.12). While cloth for the *saddetta* was first made with the heavy, sack-like cottonade, today it is made of manufactured white or off-white cotton cloth called *abu jedid* (Arabic for 'of the new') or *mamuudi* made in textile factories in Addis Ababa and Dire Dawa. The dress is no longer wound tightly across the breast with the ends hidden. Instead, the cloth is secured at the waist with *sabbata* and at the shoulder with a final tie (Figure 2.13). This style allows the cloth to drape loosely across the torso and back but keeps the sides exposed to allow for nursing, and creates a storage space for small objects at the waist. Owing to the complex folding and tucking, all the *saddetta* styles, whether they are made from one piece of fabric or two, appear to be visually constructed of two pieces of cloth. This directly mimics the leather skirt and cloth wrapper worn when cloth was first incorporated into the women's ensemble of dress.

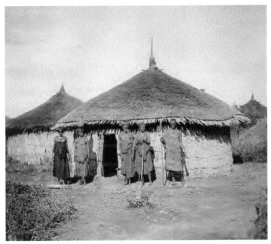

2.10 Women wearing Saddetta in a Compound (Source: Paulitschke 1888a, 31)

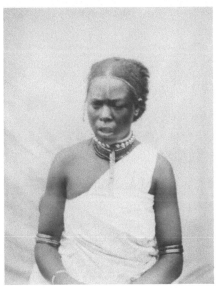

2.11. Young Afran Qallo Woman (Source: Paulitschke 1888a, 24)

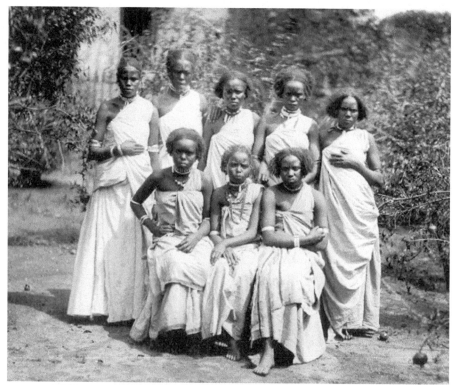

2.12   *Young Afran Qallo Women (Source: Paulitschke 1888a, 28F)*

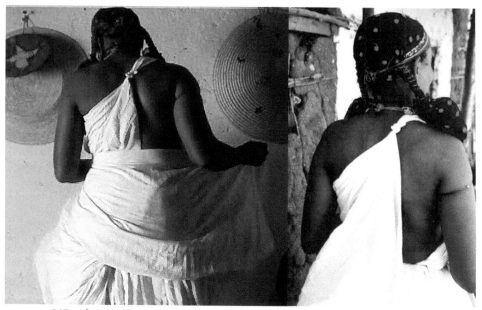

2.13   *Afran Qallo Woman wearing Gufta Hairnet Wrapping the Saddetta*

The space created by the folds of the *saddetta* at the stomach when wearing *qaxaamursa* is referred to as '*goosha*', that is, a place to privately carry valuables. Indeed, women will place material goods within this hidden space, but it is also meant to shield the stages of pregnancy from view. Since many Oromo women work in the markets in and around Harar, selling wood, coal, *khat* or foodstuffs, they must often travel along paths where they may confront foreigners; harmful animals, such as snakes and hyenas; and possessing and harm-inflicting spirits that reside close to springs and road crossings. Women say that their wrapped *saddetta* allows them to protect their bodies, particularly the region of the belly, not only from the elements but also from spiritually dangerous encounters. Women soaked the white cottonade in butter, milk, and/or a clay slip as they had done to their leather dress. Kabir notes that this was done not only to soften the material, but to protect the wearer from negative forces in the environment. In this sense, women transformed the new cotton material into something familiar and talismanic.

While Oromo men close to Harar were trading in cloth and probably wearing mostly cotton textiles at least by the mid-eighteenth century, the women's *saddetta* is distinct in design and arrangement on the body from the men's cloth *tobe*s or *chuchu* (*huchu*). The *saddetta* is also visually distinct from the dress of neighboring Amhara, Harari, and Argobba women. This resistance to cloth until the time of the Egyptian Occupation and the conservative approach to stylistic innovation still practiced today suggest the importance of the decorated female body in creating a distinctive Oromo historical identity. When forced to wear cloth, women manipulated it in such a way as to resemble the cut and folds of the leather predecessors.

The cloth wrapper embraced by Oromo women after 1875 has remained stylistically consistent over the last 150 years, and it is symbolically connected to the gradual disintegration of pastoralism for the sedentary life of agriculture and trade, and the gradual exchange of traditional political and religious institutions for Islam and foreign rule. The fact that this dress, in style and its folds, has survived through the Egyptian upheaval and the ensuing incorporation of Harar into the Ethiopian empire suggests that a woman's decorated body serves as a vehicle through which the past can be selectively invoked, particularly at moments of crisis when identity is called into question.

Transformations in Jewelry

The main commercial thoroughfare within Jugal (the local term for the walled city of Harar) is today peppered with jewelry stores. Harar is renowned in Ethiopia for its smithing families who produced high-quality silver pieces decorated with filigree and appliqué, and who, more often today, create gold jewelry of superior craftsmanship. On special occasions, affluent women who still possess these family treasures or their modern replicas made of copper, nickel, brass or aluminum, wear cylindrical metal containers called '*wakari*', hollow, granulated silver bead necklaces called '*muriyya*', and metal chain headpieces with five or seven suspended chain triangles called '*qarmaa looti*' or '*siyassa*' (Figures 2.14, 2.15,

2.16). These objects, especially those of finer quality, such as the *siyassa* forehead band, bear direct correspondence to Arabic sources introduced at the time of the Egyptian Occupation. They share much in common with silverwork from North Africa and the Middle East.

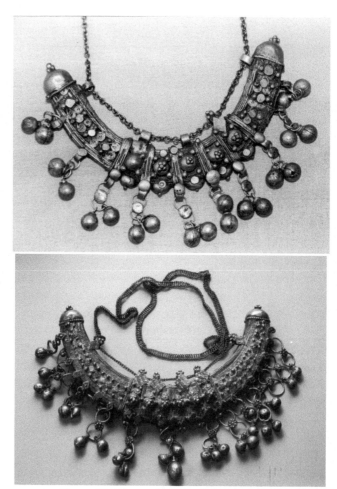

Figure 2.14 Examples of Wakari Necklaces

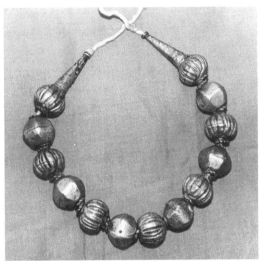

Figure 2.15 Muriyya Necklace

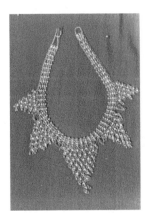
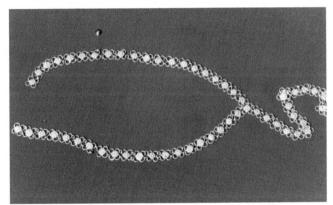

Figure 2.16 Silver Headbands Qarmaa Looti and Siyassa

Informants from smithing families living east of Jarso explain that in the late sixteenth or early seventeenth century (the time of Tabo Mormo), Arab traders with whom the Oromo traded in gum, taught their forefathers how to smelt iron and how to fashion farming and herding implements (J.A., M.A., February 3, 2000; A.A.J., May 16, 2010).[27] Before this time, the Oromo probably bartered animal products for weapons, and tools produced by Harari smiths. From Burton's description, it is assumed that women, who were wearing leather dresses at this time, were creating jewelry with natural materials of leather, shells, horn, seeds, and grasses:

> The ear is decorated with . . . red coral beads, the neck with necklaces of the same material, and the forearms with six or seven of the broad circles of buffalo and other dark horns prepared in Western India. Finally, stars are tattooed on the bosom, the eyebrows are lengthened with dyes, the eyes fringed with Kohl, and the hands and feet stained with henna. (Burton 1987, 17)

By the early nineteenth century, however, the caravan trade through the Ogaden handled by Somali middlemen brought a regular supply of iron to the Oromo with which they fashioned tools, weapons, and women's jewelry (Paulitschke 1888a, 39). In addition, the markets in Harar were, under the Egyptians, flooded with coins, including the Maria Theresa thaler, the Egyptian piaster, the rupien, and, on occasion, the locally produced mahalaq from the days of the emirs. Each coin, in turn, made its way into Oromo, Abyssinian, Argobba, and Somali costumes of the time. The Maria Theresa thaler, a silver coin with the portrait of the Austro-Hungarian Queen and a minting date of 1780, has remained the main source of silver for jewelry and other decorations throughout the eastern Highlands (Figure 2.17). Young Alla, Nole, and Jarso women began wearing silver bracelets called 'gummee' and 'girja' (Figure 2.18). *Girja* is the thick silver armband worn just above the elbow, while *gummee* is usually a thinner silver bracelet that decorates the wrist. Older Oromo women state that these bracelets replaced the *meedicha* (leather bracelets) they wore when leather skirts adorned their bodies (A.A.J., April 4, 2000; M. M. March 5, 2000). Just as imported cloth came to replace the leather dress, metal armbands took the place of leather wristbands and armbands under Egyptian governance.

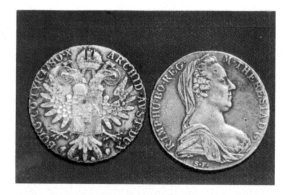

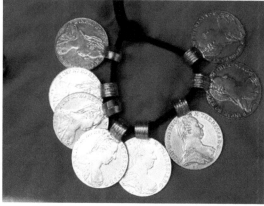

2.17 The Maria Theresa Thaler and Replicas from Wallo

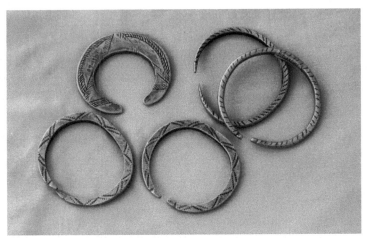

2.18 Gummee Bracelets

Necklaces also transformed from shell, rock, teeth, bone, and clay beads on leather and giraffe hair cords to metal pennant cases. Pennant cases were made up of thin sheets of pounded silver with a central pocket to contain Qur'anic verses or medicinal plants. Some construction techniques, curvilineal patterns, and dangling attachment suggest Yemeni origins. The influx of Yemeni metallurgists to Harar in the last quarter of the nineteenth century brought filigree and repoussé designs from the Arab world, and these designs continue to influence metalwork today (Figure 2.19). Hollow silver bells, which are attached to cases, bracelets, anklets, belts and necklaces, came originally from Narjan in southern Saudi Arabia and were taken up with zeal as a decorative feature among the Oromo as they had with Bedouins throughout the Islamic world (Ross 1989: 66). Burton (1987, 181), describing a woman's necklace called '*jilbah*' or '*kardas*' on the road from Marar Prairie to Harar, states that the piece is "a string of little silver bells and other ornaments made by the Arabs at Berberah."

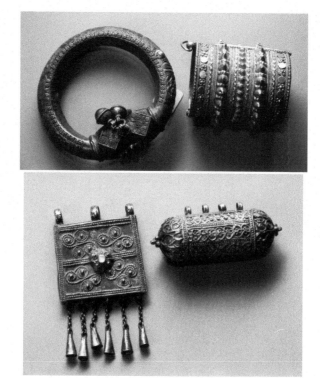

Figure 2.19 Metalwork with Yemini Influence created by Harari Smiths

The great decrease in silverwork after the time of Paulitschke may reflect the fact that extreme taxes were levied on local people at the time of the Egyptian Occupation. When the Egyptians pulled out of Harar, not only were local people forced to surrender large amounts of currency and agricultural surplus, but the Egyptians are said to have taken sacks of Maria Theresa coins with them. An Afran Qallo men's song recorded in a village in Fedis mentions the Egyptian taking of silver:

> The sack of coffee is taken to one's house,
> The silver that is loved is taken overseas.
> You tied beads together for your forehead,
> One is interlocked with another.
> And you tied your stomach with cloth,
> But my head and stomach are shaking for you.[28]

In this passage, a man sings about the beloved silver carried away by Egyptian officials. He also mentions the beaded forehead ornament that comes to replace *siyassa* (and is still worn today). Lastly, he sings about her *sabbatta*, bound around her stomach and, in contrast, his shaking stomach analogous to her containment and his wildness.

Another Oromo song about the Egyptian period suggests the political upheaval experienced by the inhabitants, as well as the silver and gold to which the singer is comparing his love. The song discusses the Oromo *kilkillee* (silver bracelet), and the silver and gold hoop earring known as '*looti*':

> Harar is full of people and there is a mob.
> Even the ground itself shakes.
> Look, *kilkillee* on her arm and *looti* on her head.
> In this Jijjiga area, there is a place called Haroo Cinaaksanii.
> If the area is to go to war, there is chaos.
> You are numerous kinds of gold with melting silver.[29]

If silver coins left Harar around 1885, fine jewelry making must have been on the decline. Certainly, by the time of King Menelik's annexation of Harar, many women report that their mothers and grandmothers had sold off their *girja* and *gummee* or given them to Harari smiths to melt into headbands. The metal headbands, known as '*qarmaa looti*', are one of the few silver items that some agricultural Oromo families living outside the wall still own today. Those who cannot afford it, use low-grade metal spooling or, in the last decade, imported seed beads.

Though harder to find, the Maria Theresa thaler has remained the main source of silver for jewelry and other decorations throughout Ethiopia. It was no longer allowed to be imported or exported after 1933, when the Bank of Ethiopia issued its own paper notes and coin. The thaler has taken on a second career as a necklace centerpiece throughout Ethiopia or as the supplier of silver for other ornaments.

During the Egyptian Occupation of Harar, metal headbands, necklaces and armband replaced the natural beads strung on leather popular during Burton's time. When the Egyptians depleted the supply of precious metals upon their departure, Oromo women turned to newly arrived, mass-produced materials, including the rubber armbands, industrial metal spooling, and seed beads, which they still use today and which is discussed further in the final chapter of this book. The silver ornaments that some family members were able to retain have become symbols of the Egyptian period, a time of chaos and strife. Today, they play a prominent, homeopathic role in warding off dangerous forces in the environment, including negative spirits, wild animals, and strangers with harmful intent. Shiny metal pieces also play a central role in women's spirit possession ceremonies discussed in Chapter 5. In both cases, older arm and torso jewelry of silver, and more recent metal imitations, especially those that hold talismanic materials, are used to reflect danger and allude to subjugation under Egyptian rule.

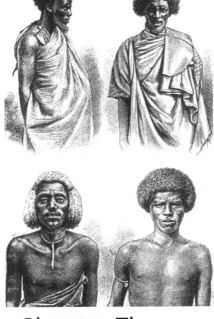

Chapter Three

Tying Oromo History

The Manipulation of Dress during the Time of Menelik

The Oromo describe their forefathers' and foremothers' relationships with the ethnic groups and ruling dynasties of Harar and its regions as constantly fluctuating. Long before the Egyptian Occupation of Harar (1875–1885) that preceded the Abyssinian invasion, each Oromo *gosa* (clan) placed these neighbors into one of three categories that determined who they considered hostile and with whom they would collaborate at different moments. For each, the body could be dressed to illustrate that specific relationship. The first category, *warra* (family) is designated for those with whom one shares *gosa* blood or those who have been adopted into the *gosa*. The Oromo regard the few emirs of Harar with whom they swore an oath of brotherhood as *fira* (relatives), thereby creating a binding support network. It was common for Oromo clans who shared a *fira* bond with the emir to demand from him goods and financial support in exchange for familial allegiances. The second relational category is *amba* (community). *Amba* consists of those with whom one trades, works, and occasionally marries but who are not blood relations or enemies. The emirs and other leaders who took Oromo spouses or married their offspring into Oromo families, and those who developed trade between the walled city of Harar and Oromo communities were considered, along with their family and followers, *amba*. This bond was largely based on economic exchange. Finally, the last designated relationship is *diina* (enemy). *Diina* is further divided into two meanings. One refers to those groups with whom the Oromo were at war in the past but whom they have not fought within several generations and with whom, like many Somali clans, they may intermarry. Some Oromo place the Egyptian rulers in this category. *Diina* may also mean those who are characterized as perpetual enemies, who deceive, wound and kill without mercy and who will even target individuals considered sanctified by Oromo law, namely Oromo women, children and the elderly. This latter type of *diina* violates the sacred, breaks all conventions of war, and it is of the gravest offense.

Each relationship described above was recorded and passed on to subsequent generations by Oromo oral historians who, along with the political and military council leaders of *raba-dori*, proscribed the appropriate course of action. As far as dress is concerned, men and women used their adornment to indicate particular states of allegiances. Dress, particularly the dress of women in the case of the *diina* relationship, was tactically used by men to solicit the sympathies of the enemy groups, particularly when peace offerings were to be presented by the offending party in order to re-establish harmonious relations. On some occasions from the 1890s onward, warriors would take off their headpieces and put down their weapons in order to wear the central component of a married woman's costume, her *saddetta* (white cotton dress) and/or her *guftaa (*black hairnet) (see Figure 2.12). The wearing of *saddetta* and *guftaa* was intended to communicate submission, humility, and concurrence after a period of aggression and the loss of life. The following three examples illustrate how the dress of a woman, when worn by a man, serves as a visual oath for peace.[30] These examples counter those of women dressing in men's combat attire to follow.

Oromo elders state that when council leaders went to Walaabu each year to see the Abba Muuda (father of anointment), the *raba-dori* ritual leader who guarded Oromo law, those who "carried the spoken law," dressed in a woman's traditional dress, *saddetta*. These men would wrap eight yards of sheeting around their torso and tie the ends over their right shoulder intending to show that while they were frail and could no longer fight, they nevertheless carried within them broad knowledge of the Oromo constitution. In this sense, a woman's dress suggested that these men were to be respected not for their physical prowess which had long since deteriorated, but for the wisdom that came with old age. Secondly, in the 1970s, the sixty-five-year-old Afran Qallo *heera* (Oromo law) leader Adam Wadaayi placed a woman's *guftaa* on his head as he walked to meet his *gosa* near Dire Dawa (S.M.G., July 23, 2004). Someone from his *gosa* had killed someone from another *gosa*, and since the individual could not pay the *guma* or blood money, he traveled to his *gosa* head to ask for help. He tied *guftaa* around his hair in order to placate the angry family of the deceased and to renew peaceful relations. In this guise he was successful in begging the *gosa* leaders to provide the obligatory animals of retribution for the deceased's clan.

A final example comes from the Kundhublee, a subclan of the Nole *gosa*. The Kundhublee have a long history of feuding with the Issa Somali. In the 1940s, the Nole war leader, Buraalee Sarsaree, donned a woman's *guftaa* (hairnet)while talking to the assembly of Nole clan leaders (M.S.S., March 3, 2000).[31] The wearing of this garment was intended to instill patience and restraint in his followers as they plotted how to mobilize against the enemy. After this meeting, the Nole warriors successfully pushed the Issa through the semi-desert along the rail tracks to Djibouti.

In each of these cases, the wearing of a married woman's dress or hairnet came to embody a plea for leniency, patience, and peace. Older women also recalled the oaths that they took to maintain peace when their mothers covered their hair with the *guftaa* netting for the first time. Indeed, it is the tying of these garments that is said secure peaceful action in the wearer. It is clear that Oromo women's dress and what women wear convey proper codes of conduct, specifically during states of unrest.

Despite donning a woman's *guftaa*, men's attempts to placate the Shawa invaders of the late 1800s proved futile. The conflict with Menelik's forces is mentioned by elders as the most barbaric encounter in the collective consciousness of the Oromo people. Warriors quickly became aware that these enemies would not succumb to their usual protocols for peace and a *diina* relationship formed (A.Y. February 20, 2000; S.M.G. July 25, 2004). The stage was set for all-out warfare and women, who were customarily restricted from battle, fought with men. Their participation in the rebellion against Menelik's troops and the large loss of life sustained by the Barentuma Oromo, became the impetus for a change in women's dress. In this case, the women who survived began to wear specific articles of dress associated with war during and after the infiltration of the Abyssinian soldiers in order to convey their hostile *diina* relationship with these foreigners. Oromo women successfully communicated this through their increased visibility and movement as travelers and traders.

In 1885, the Mahdist revolt in the Sudan forced the Egyptians to abandon Harar and the Egyptian Pasha and British consul placed on the throne, Emir Abdullahi Ali Abd al-Shakur (1885–1887), the last ruler of the independent city-state. He ruled with an eye toward isolating the town from intruders, including the Oromo, who were perceived as threatening to his dominion. During this time, many of the traders and entrepreneurs involved in commerce who had settled in Harar left for the coast. As a result, the Oromo presence around the immediate vicinity of the walled city grew stronger (Paulitschke 1888b, 208). The presence of women was especially prominent. An estimated two-thirds of the entire Harar population in 1885 consisted of women, a fact that Philipp Paulitschke (1888b, 208) suggests was equally true on the outskirts of the city where mainly Oromo resided.[32]

The reasons for the enhanced visibility of women are likely connected to the following four points. First, the strong agricultural business that had grown up among the Oromo communities outside the wall had been established largely by women. While most Oromo men within a sixty-mile radius of the city had adopted farming as a full-time profession, women traveled to trade their agricultural surpluses in the Harar markets. While special markets for the exchange of livestock were controlled and frequented by men, they existed primarily in neighboring Oromo regions such as Fedis. Oromo women, however, walked weekly to and from the countryside to the Harar market, where they would have been more visible to foreigners such as Paulitschke. Second, this period of growing isolationism saw a decline in the merchant economy as foreign traders deserted the town and Emir Abdullahi Ali Abd al-Shakur reclaimed the age-old institution of slavery. In 1885 he attacked the surrounding Oromo villages and sold the male captives to slavers heading toward the coast (Shell, M.S.S., March 3, 2000). Paulitschke (1888b, 261) mentions that while he was in Harar, the slavers fled with "[Oromo] to smuggle them into the city and take them with a caravan to Zeila and Berbera." Coupled with the killings at the hands of the Somali, the emirs, or other *diina* groups, there were literally fewer Oromo men around. Third, it was in 1885 that the *abba bokkus*, the *raba-dori* leaders, began to practice publicly again and the institution of *raba-dori* was reinstated (Paulitschke 1888b, 313). Men were spending a great deal of time undercover trying to restore the generational grade system, perform vital ceremonies, and create new laws, all of which had been put on hold for the ten years of Egyptian sovereignty. Fourth, reports had already been filtering into Harar that Menelik, King of Shawa, had crossed into the Awash Valley and had ordered his troops to destroy Ittu Oromo groups they met on the road to Harar in an attempt to bring under control the land and the Oromo themselves (Caulk 1971, 10; Paulitschke 1888b, 197). Fearing that their own land and lives might next be in jeopardy, men might have been directing their attention to the formation of defensive strategies in private settings. For these reasons, Oromo women were more visible than ever before. It was at this time, with Egyptian laws on dress no longer in place and Oromo men's attentions diverted due to the slaughter sustained under Menelik, that women's dress becomes a prominent political statement. In particular, the tying of fiber and leather to the body signals the displacement, enslavement, and bloodshed experienced by the Oromo community during this period.[33]

Menelik: Men's *Harrii* in Place of Women's *Sabbata*

As previously discussed, a cloth waist sash called 'sabbata,' has traditionally been used to harness a married women's dress of white sheeting, *saddetta*, at the waist (see Figure 2.6). As a marker of marriage, it is an important symbol of womanhood for its connections to fertility, land, and history. As mentioned above, oral history speaks of the Great Oromo mother, the primordial mother of all Oromo people, tying this belt during the great Barentuma migration. As she encircled her waist with eight yards of cloth, she bequeathed land to her eight grandsons, and in the repetition of this gesture, each succeeding generation recognizes the historical role women played in law and governance within *raba-dori* as they repeat this action.

When a woman's mother first binds the *sabbata* around her daughter's waist at marriage, she reminds her daughter of this important legend. In general, the *sabbata* has come to stand for the peace, patience, and security associated with motherhood. However, during the time of the Menelik's invasion, this changed. This emblem of peace was removed and replaced with a men's fiber belt. Oromo female elders I spoke with in 2000 remember stories of their foremothers participating as soldiers and spies in the struggle against the invading Abyssinian army. In one particularly vivid account, women climbed the mountains Tulluu Gambisaa, Tulluu Barruu, and Tulluu Ijaa and tied cowhides to the trees. They beat the skins with sticks in order to sound an alert to Oromo forces that foreign soldiers were coming so that the men might prepare defensive strategies. Those women who were captured by Menelik's forces in the act of sounding the alarm were marched to Anollee in Arsi. There, many were mutilated or killed (A.Y., February 20, 2004). In 2014, the Annolee Martys Memorial Monument was unveiled, a severed hand holding a severed breast, to commemorate "fallen mothers and fathers" and their brutal treatment on the battlefield (Figure 3.1). During their participation in the war, these heroic women who gave their lives are said to have taken off their *sabbata* as emblems of peace and replaced them with *harrii*. The *harrii*, a reed waist piece plaited for young men by women, had previously been worn during the *raba-dori* generational-grade period of warriorhood and served as a receptacle for weapons. Both *raba-dori*, which had been outlawed during the Egyptian Occupation, and the fiber belts, during Menelik's invasion, were no longer in use. Remembered and recounted by the Afran Qallo today, this act, the removal of the *sabbata* and the tying of *harrii*, aroused strong Oromo nationalist sentiment during the conquest and colonization of the Oromo. The gesture not only signified the state of war and the presence of the enemy, but also alerted the broader Oromo community that women, who traditionally served as agents for harmonious relations, were now actively engaged in combat with men. While this act was short lived, it signals the significant role dress played during this experience.

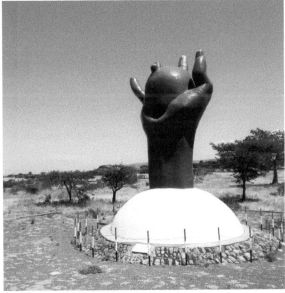

Figure 3.1 The Annolee Martys Memorial Monument. A Severed Hand holding a Severed Breast

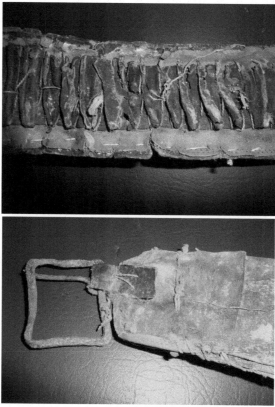

Figure 3.2 The Sinnaara Belt used to hold Ammunition

After this period, the wearing of *sabbata* resumed and was again associated with a peaceful state of being. Informants told me that today daughters are taught to bind the *sabbata* tightly as a means of symbolically binding, and thus ensuring, peaceful relations. In this sense, the *sabbata* as a symbol of peace is intended to serve as a kind of talisman to ward off periods of *diina* warfare associated with *harrii*. *Harrii* as a sign of warriorhood, first for men during *raba-dori* and later for women during Menelik's invasion, is also connected to the modern belts called *sinnaara* used to hold ammunition (Figure 3.2). Oromo men had been acquiring guns since the first decades of the twentieth century. After their initial defeat against Menelik's forces on January 7, 1887 at the Battle of Calanqoo, thirty-seven miles from Harar, and many subsequent battles with Abyssinian troops, Oromo men fashioned *sinnaara* (bullet holsters) to wear around their waists. Women created a song at this time that compares the *harrii* that their foremothers once wore to the *sinnaara* that men adopted:

> In the springtime, the Baali leaves blossoms
> So how's the sinaara faring, having replaced the harrii?[34]

Herein, the singer inquires after the condition of the Oromo during the great turmoil of the coming of Menelik when the *raba-dori* governing system, represented in men's belts, was completely replaced with the rule of foreign weapons, represented by the foreign bullet holster. The *sinnaara,* then, is an icon of modern warfare. This item of dress continues to be worn today by men and women who participate in the Ethiopian National Defense Force or as freedom fighters. While it no longer resembles the reed belt that men and a few women warriors once wore, the *sinnaara* today is emblematic of the challenges Oromo soldiers faced in the late 19th century.

Men's Dress and the Reign of Emperor Menelik (1889–1913)

During the Battle of Calanqoo, nearly 4,000 Oromo and Harari soldiers under the Emir fought Menelik's 30,000 troops (Rimbaud 1887). The French poet Rimbaud, (1887) who was trading armaments in the region, reports:

> The engagement scarcely lasted a quarter of an hour . . . Three thousand warriors were cut up with sabers and crushed in a blink of an eye by the King of Shoa. Nearly 200 Sudanese, Egyptians, and Turcs left with Abdullaï after the Egyptian evacuation, and perished with the Galla and Somali warriors. This is why it is said that when the Shoan soldiers (who have never killed any whites) returned, they brought back from Harar the testicles of foreigners.

Mohammed Hassen (1980, 244) also reports that the Oromo of Harar "say among those who participated in the battle, none came back without losing either a hand or a leg or penis." Arsi and Ittu women, who also participated on the battlefront as Menelik marched east, did not fare much better. Informants state that among the Arsi Oromo to the southwest of Harar, Menelik's soldiers mutilated women who participated in the fighting by cutting off their right hand, left leg, and/or right breast (S.R. April 4, 2000). Martial De Salviac (1901, 350), a French missionary, who lived among the Oromo during this time, states that among the Arsi Oromo "the right wrist of 400 notable Oromo [were cut] in one day alone. We have seen with our own eyes some of these glorious ones mutilated." Harming women in this manner was subject to very severe penalties according to *heera*, Oromo law. If the right breast is cut or severed, the breast from which babies most frequently drink, the guilty party must pay the equivalent of one human life.[35] Without her right breast, a new mother's babies are more likely to die. The fact that economic retribution was denied to the families of the thousands of Oromo men and women killed or harmed in attacks by Menelik's army permanently sealed the invaders as *diina*. These aggressors were, according to the traditions of *heera*, placed into the second categorical distinction of *diina,* a relationship of eternal enemies beyond the reach of reconciliation who target members of society who legally must remain unharmed: women, children, and the elderly.

After his victory, King Menelik's soldiers entered Harar and immediately took possession of the settlements owned by the families of those warriors who had been defeated in the Battle of Calanqoo. As a punishment for their resistance, households in the city and the surrounding villages were also fined between 50,000 and 75,000 silver thalers (Hassen 1980, 235). Further, when Menelik returned to Shawa, the Gondari, the nickname of the soldiers left behind in Harar, "resorted to open brigandage, raiding and looting the countryside" (236). The years following the influx of the Abyssinians into Harar were particularly challenging to the Afran Qallo, since over 12,000 Abyssinian soldiers and their families and slaves relied for their survival on the tribute and taxes from Oromo communities. Oromo men who did not comply with paying the heavy taxes were dragged by mules. Women could at any moment be forced into servitude, required to use their own grain to make bread for the soldiers and their families, fetch water for them, and bring them firewood. Rimbaud (1887), while in Harar, writes:

> Collecting taxes in the surrounding region only happens through raids, in which villages are burned, livestock is stolen, and populations are taken away in slavery. The revenue from the [Oromo], customs, trading posts, markets, and other receipts, are stolen by anyone who can get at the . . . Ménélik completely lacks funds, always remaining in the most complete ignorance of (or indifference to) the exploitation of the region's resources, which he has forced into submission. He only thinks about accumulating guns in order to allow himself to send his troops to levy men from the [Oromo].

Driven by this persistent plundering, many Oromo families ceased farming communally and stopped their participation in trade with the coast. In the years to follow, the land tenure system imposed by Menelik forced the Oromo to convert remaining farmland to coffee plantations for exportation. The growing of the *khat* crop was also launched as a cash crop.[36] Despite these changes in land rights, the Oromo remained deeply invested in their land. When Ras Makonnen, Menelik's governor of Harar province and the father of the future Ethiopian emperor Haile Selassie, embarked on a road-building project through Oromo land using Oromo laborers this was aptly recorded. Robert Skinner (quoted in Pankhurst 1975, 2), the first U.S. envoy to Ethiopia, published the alleged conversations between the Afran Qallo and Ras Makonnen:

> When the fine new highway was projected between Dire-Daouah and Harrar, it became necessary to condemn the land required for its construction. The Gallas waited upon Ras Makonnen, their Governor. Their farms would be ruined, they said; the work <u>must</u> not go on: they could not accept the price offered for their land.

> 'But it is a good, fair price, is it not?' Said the Ras.

> 'It is not the price we complain of, most gracious lord; we don't want our farms to be destroyed.'

> The Ras ordered them out of his presence, saying that there was but one
> Governor of Harar, and that he and he alone would say what might or might
> not be done. The road was constructed, and a guard prevented interference
> with the labourers.

As land was taken, farmers and their families were forced into tenancy as tribute-paying subjects (*gabbar*). As livelihoods and land were destroyed, other lifeways were being eroded. By 1900, Menelik had banned all meetings of the *raba-dori* assembly (*chafe*), prayer gatherings, and the celebrated pilgrimage to the land of Abba Muuda in southern Ethiopia (Knutsson 1967, 155). The institution of Abba Muuda, the celebrated Oromo ritual leader, had served for generations as the focal point of pan-Oromo unity (Greenfield and Hassen 1992, 577). Without these cultural and religious practices, the Oromo were left with only Islam as a legitimate organizing ideology. Mohammed Hassen (2000, 101) writes:

> Deprived of their freedom and political institutions, reduced to the status of
> landless *gabbars* in their own land, the Oromo of Hararghe had no choice
> but to look to Islam to provide them with an ideological framework and
> institutional expression in order to survive the shock of violent defeat, loss
> of land, destruction of their political, cultural and religious institutions,
> dehumanization, subjugation and economic exploitation. It was this situation
> which appears to have turned them to Islam *en masse*, as a form of rejection of
> the colonial order created by Emperor Menilek.

As more and more Oromo turned to Islam as a new, legitimate, non-threatening, and non-colonial organizing principle, they adopted Muslim dress as well. However, while men adopted the imported cloth waist wraps and collared dress shirts that left them indistinguishable from their Muslim Harari, Somali, and Argobba neighbors, Oromo women maintained their *saddetta*, adding only a head scarf in public as a sign of their new religious identity. Oromo women's bodies remained a visual connection to the pre-colonial period. This is most readily apparent among pastoralist communities who were more erratically mistreated by the Abyssinian state than their agricultural counterparts. One Oromo elder recounted:

> It wasn't until the Amhara came that they tried to destroy our language, our
> dancing, and our culture. Oromo farmers were so impoverished that they hadn't
> the time or resources to recreate their traditions. Only among the pastoralists
> is a strong sense of our culture still available. A man who practiced his culture
> during the time of Menelik and Haile Sellassie was arrested, and the name of
> the crime was "*Kuburnakkaa*" ("You shamed the king"). Only women were
> left alone. (R.M.O., March 6, 2000)

While many Oromo men turned to Islam, others, particularly among more urban populations, began adopting an Abyssinian/Amhara-centered identity. Along with the acceptance of Amhara cultural practices, name changes, and the use of the Amharic language, Abyssinian ornaments provided some relief from persecution for Oromo men, even if they continued to identify as Muslims.[37] For example, by foregoing traditional forms of adornment and adopting wooden and metal neck crosses during Menelik's and later, Haile Selassie's rule, Oromo men visually showed their allegiance to the Ethiopian Orthodox Church and were therefore allowed access to some of the privileges afforded the ruling Amhara ethnic group. A Muslim Oromo man who traveled frequently to the capital and other Christian urban settlements might adopt highland Christian dress or tie on a cross and baptismal chord in order to "blend in," yet these items were tossed aside when one returned to his Muslim community (A.S.J., October 6, 1999). Donham (1986, 11) writes that "for those of the frontiers, Christian identity promised an escape from the worst aspects of Abyssinian domination."

We find then that during this time of colonization, the adoption of an Islamic or Orthodox Christian identity, whether sincere or superficial, was outwardly proclaimed through men's dress. In either case, dress became a highly calculated and communicative indicator of one's faith. Yet, despite these new dress codes for men, we find that both men and women continued to embrace a deeply significant Oromo act-that of tying leather onto the body. Pieces of leather could be wrapped around biceps, ankles, spears, and scepters without drawing much attention. Both the materials and the act of tying, however, reinforced Oromo values and offered a non-verbal code of actions of actors.

Tying *Meedicha*

A simple leather tie still used by Oromo to secure the legs of livestock, is intimately connected to the pastoral livelihood of the first ancestors. When worn by humans, these same straps of leather fashioned from hide and secured around the wrist, upper arm and neck are called *meedicha* (*maadiicha*) and are virtually indistinguishable from the *gaadi*, the leather strap that holds the milking cow's legs. Both the *gaadi* and the *meedicha* leather cord are made from a strip of the thickest skin of a cow, goat, or camel, dyed red in a mixture of boiled bark and herbs. Symbolically, both act as a marker of the value placed on pastoral livelihood. The *meedicha* mentioned by Paulitschke (1896, 279) was intended to be worn by all participants when a female animal was to be slaughtered. Today, Oromo women also wear *meedicha* tied with a piece of incense (*qumbi*) at the wrist. Like the leather of the Civet cat, who is known for its musk-like odor, the *meedicha* with incense is intended to ward off *buda*, those with the evil eye. The idea of *buda*, a foreign concept prior to colonization, resonated for the Oromo as the embodiment of the danger of foreigners from whom they sought to protect themselves through adornment. The modern leather bracelet strung with incense is efficacious not as a visual deflector like most talismans, but rather for its pungent smell. Those with the evil eye are said to be repulsed by the odor and flee. During the time of Menelik's colonization, however, *meedicha* become a symbol of men and women's active participation in warfare.

The *meedicha* has several symbolic associations that relate to specific historical periods. For example, only one generation ago, *meedicha*, tied on the left wrist, indicated a woman's status as single; when tied on the right wrist, proclaimed her engagement; when tied on the upper arm, indicated her status as married. If worn by a well-respected woman during the time of *raba-dori* in conjunction with her *siqqee* or *lookkoo*, (wooden scepter), it communicated not only her power but her sacrality. A physical or verbal attack made against her while she carried these items was tantamount to war.

For young men during the time of *raba-dori*, *meedicha* worn on the neck, both wrists and upper arm showed a man's status as a hero. The number of pieces he wore at each site is indicative of the number of lives taken either with his weapons or with his own hands. Female warriors also wore *meedicha* to show their status as killers, but they wore the leather tied on the forehead, called *dhihee*, accompanied by an ostrich feather. If a female warrior merely maimed or cut someone, the leather tie encircled her ankle. To show that her father, brother, and husband were warriors, she wore *meedicha* on her upper arm.

In each of these cases, *meedicha* can function as a metonym for the protective power of the slaughtered animal or the death of an enemy. During the rule of Menelik, informants state that the *meedicha* was worn by both men and women for its talismanic capacity in the face of much anxiety (M.R.A., February 20, 2000). The most potent leather from which to make *meedicha* during the reign of Menelik came from the dried skin of the horses used by his Amhara soldiers (S.M.G., February 25, 2000). In this sense, the destructive ability of the horse and rider is harnessed in the leather tie in much the same way that the *sabbata* is used to keep out potential harm and propagate harmonious relations.

While the *meedicha* necklace was still being worn during Menelik's reign, a time when clothing of cotton weave had already replaced women's soft leather dresses, it has fallen into disuse today in favor of other types of necklaces, alerting us to the fact that fashion, no less than identity, is always in a state of flux.

During the late nineteenth century, women revived a historic item of men's dress associated with violence and tied it in place of the *sabbata*. The wearing of *harrii* was later replaced with *sinnaara* by men and less frequently by women. Whether wearing *harrii, sabbata* or *meedicha* made from the skin of the enemy's horse, dress is tied onto the body. This tying is a deliberate act intended to secure the doctrine of war on the body, to prepare and protect it from danger, and to alert others to one's intent. Even as new materials, colors, and forms continue to change dress styles for men and women today, the act of tying continues to seal and conceal that which is most revered.

Women describe this historical period in which their foremothers became warriors as a time of great violence and chaos (Z.A., February 20, 2000; M.R.A., February 20, 2000; R.M.O., March 6, 2000). After all, an Oromo proverb states: While the father is a tree outside, the mother is the center-post for the house.[38] Women were expected to maintain peace and uphold stable relations. With the influx of social, political, religious, and economic changes brought about during the Egyptian presence and the Abyssinian invasion of Oromo lands, women's dress and what women wore was strategically used to signal hostile relationships. The use of fiber and leather bindings by Oromo women became markers of war and proper action during the conquest and colonization of their homeland near the city-state of Harar under Menelik, King of Shawa, in the late 1880s.[39] *Harrii* (the waist belt) and *meedicha* (the leather tie) became symbols of the crisis brought about by the Abyssinian invasion, and when tied around the body today, these objects activate collective memories of these experiences.

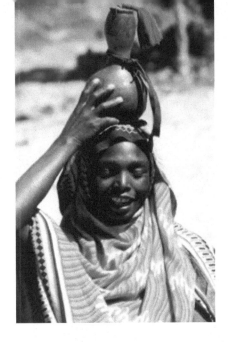

Chapter Four

Women's Bodies and Women's Rights in Oromo Law

The tying of leather or cloth at the waist for the Afran Qallo is symbolic of fecundity and historical experience. The opposite motion, that of cutting the body as a way of mutilation, also plays a pivotal role in Oromo thought. This chapter examines the way the female body is considered and protected in terms of disfigurement and violence.

During the time prior to the Egyptian Occupation, Afran Qallo Oromo women's public participation in the traditional governing system *raba-dori* was limited to the role of observer, witness, and ritual sponsor. They were not policymakers or decision makers, but their bodies could become the visual marker for the generational grades of their fathers, brothers, and husbands. Usually living outside the domain of their father's clan after marriage, they did not enter elderhood grades with their male counterparts. Even after menopause when women in some east African societies could take on leadership roles typically aligned with men, Oromo women were excluded from public political careers. Who, then, protects a woman's rights? Largely, women's own religious and social institutions guard women's bodies and well-being supported by the Oromo constitution. Oromo law is so specific in terms of the female body that the subject warrants a closer examination of women's bodies, women's judicial staffs, and power relations within Oromo society.

Today, Oromo law can be challenged by local courts that often adhere to Shari'a law or the Ethiopian constitution. When I visited the town of Baabile in 1999, I found a young woman of about fifteen years in tears at the local police office (where I was required to register in order to get clearance to talk to a group of famers). I asked what had happened. This young woman explained that she had been abducted a week earlier and forced to marry a man she did not like. She burned down the thatched roof kitchen of their house and ran away. Her in-laws caught her and were now pressing charges. Through sobs she explained that this would not happen if his family had followed *heera* (Oromo traditional laws).

Heera (or *Heera Gosa*)[40] the Oromo traditional constitution, is an elaborate judiciary oral document that consists of a complex network of *seera* (laws) among and between various *gosa* (clans). In *heera*, guidelines for proper behavior and action oversaw and continue to influence some aspects of life for Barentuma Oromo. Included for women are even full sets of recipes for mixing milk, churning butter, and preparing grains to avoid inadvertently poisoning their husbands and children.

Innumerable laws within *heera* reflect the worth of a woman's body as described by elders in Baabile, Fedis, Dire Dawa, Alem Maya, and Wallo. In *heera* anything that deliberately takes away from a women's beauty through physical disfigurement and discomfort is regarded as criminal; for example, to disfigure a woman results in a fine of cattle of half *guma* or half the worth of a human life. If she is engaged, the cattle are given to her fiancé to compensate for her lack of beauty. Once her fiancé takes the cattle and marries her, he is forbidden to insult his wife's beauty and discuss her deformity in the future without punishment.

Ridiculing a woman's appearance also has judicial consequences. For any man to insult a woman because she is physically disfigured, including the loss of an eye or tooth, could result in a public flogging, a public apology, and the presentation of two or three calabashes of honey or butter and *uwa* (tanned leather) to the woman. If he continues to pester her with insults, his arms are bound behind his back and a drum is tied to his back. In humiliation, children beat the drum while they lead him around the village (an identical punishment for a crime of theft). Even worse, if a man severs parts of a woman's body, the following penalties could apply: the loss of a thumb is a fine of fifteen cows; the loss of a forefinger, six cows; middle finger, four cows; ring finger, three cows; and a pinky, two cows. While the number of cattle is based on the Nole *heera* and is therefore approximate since it may change from one region to the next, the value ratio of fingers to thumb is fixed among all Afran Qallo. The loss of a woman's eye requires a payment of fifty cows. If her right breast is cut, the breast from which babies most frequently drink, the guilty party must pay the equivalent of one human life. If a man breaks a woman's leg and it does not heal properly, he pays twenty-five cows. If he cuts her hair, he is fined ten cows. The value placed on unblemished skin is well illustrated in the Oromo constitution. If he injures her face and it produces a scar, he pays five cows. However, if a man wounds a woman's face severely and any of the following happens: the loss of one or both eyes, the loss of one or both ears or the loss of part of the nose, the attacker must pay the equivalent of the fine for *guma*, one human life to her *gosa*. If she is not married, he must also marry her and provide for her.

A woman's worth and success as a wife and mother are clearly dependent on her physical wholeness and beauty. If her face is made grotesque, she is less likely to enter into a marriage from which her *gosa* can prosper. The notion of disfigurement as seen with excessive *haaxixa* (facial scarring) and *tumtuu* (tattooing) (discussed in Chapter 5) is in direct opposition to ideal health and beauty standards that manifest in smooth, shiny skin. In a traditional love song sung on the eve of marriage, the bride's ideal skin is evoked: "Your mother mentioned your pale, smooth face, shook the milk and smeared you with butter." Here paleness is associated with dryness, the lack of color with the lack of luster. Through butter, the skin shines and becomes beautiful. Modern powder cosmetics, readily available in the kiosks in Harar, went largely unsold to Oromo, except to women in mourning or after childbirth, who purposely wanted to appear unattractive.

Without her right breast, a woman's babies are more likely to die. In *heera* the breast is equivalent to the penis and the same laws apply to its loss or injury. The lasting importance of the breast is clearly evident in the Annollee memorial which features a severed hand holding a woman's breast (Figure 3.1). In the case of deliberate harm to her breast, it is not the woman who receives compensation, but members of her patrilineage. Yusuf Ahmed (1960, 15) states that among the Ittu the loss of a breast or reproductive organ required twenty-five cattle as compensation. This is due to the fact that one's blood, by law, belongs to one's *gosa*. If any blood is lost, it is the *gosa* that has been symbolically violated, even if the female victim lives with the *gosa* of her husband. However, if she is married and her features are marred, it is her husband who receives collateral. This is because her body, or more specifically her procreative potential and physical beauty, becomes the property of her husband at marriage. Yet, as the following examples make clear, there are many regulations on the proper treatment of the wife, including restrictions placed on the husband's handling of his wife's body: If a wife is found to be a hermaphrodite or if she has some genital abnormality a husband may untie the *nika* (marriage), but if he kills her as a result, he must pay a fine of five cows to her *gosa*. A wife may also break *nika* with her husband if he cannot perform sex for any reason. If a man willfully forces his wife to have sex, he is punished on a continuum of severity – rape[41] outdoors on the earth is the most severe, while rape within the home on soft ground requires a lesser compensation of only a few cattle. To commit rape within one's own *gosa* brings *hodda* (shame) to the entire patrilineage, punishable by fines and a severe beating or, in the case of the rape of a mother, sister, or daughter, by death. If a man is killed while raping a woman or raping another man, the murderer is required to pay the collateral of one donkey to the rapist's *gosa*. The small payment of one donkey is considered a grave insult and reflects the dishonorable act carried out by the deceased before death.

Murdering a woman or man also encompasses a complex set of rules defined by the nature of the act. When homicide was committed, penalty was decided by *guma*, the highest form of blood compensation for murder in eastern Oromo society (Kabir 1995, 24). To disregard *guma* resulted in complete excommunication from the group. During *guma*, male elders from both groups held a meeting. The elders from the killer's family presented a burial shroud and a cow to the victim's clan to be slaughtered at the funeral. The family of the deceased asked for *raffisaa* (the first payment) from the murderer's family. At each meeting, an animal was slaughtered and divided in half. The right hoof and foreleg were presented to the killer's family, and the left leg was given to the deceased's family. The right leg was buried uneaten as a symbol of restraint. Today, *guma* varies from *gosa* to *gosa* and the number of cattle required has also shifted considerably in the last three generations. As the agriculturalist populations grew throughout Oromia, local elders modified the cattle fines to reflect the decreasing access to herds. In 1901, deSalviac, a French missionary in Harar, writes that crimes could even be paid in coins: murders were fined eighty Maria Theresa thalers for each death (Huntingford 1969, 63). Today, an average price for *guma* (the taking of a life) is twenty-five head of cattle, while in the past, the figure was closer to one hundred.

There are five types of *guma* payment for murder (with less punishment respectively): (1) killing intentionally, (2) killing by accident with witnesses, (3) killing with evidence but without witnesses, (4) killing a brother with whom one shares a biological mother and father, and (5) killing a brother with whom one shares only one parent. When the killer is not immediately known, all potential male enemies in the area are summoned. An oath is taken over a red-hot ember at sunset. Each man must pass the ember and say: "If I am guilty or I saw the killer, let my clan be destroyed like this ember." Then he urinates on the coal. The elders ask the guilty party and any eyewitnesses to come forward. If no one is found guilty and no evidence is found, the blood price is paid by the village nearest to where the murder occurred. Among the *heera* of the Baabile, if a man kills another man, no matter the reason, the killer's sister must be given to the brother of the dead man as a wife. By joining the two families through marriage, it is said that revenge can be avoided. If an enemy is killed, no *guma* is paid. A woman, however, even as a daughter, sister, wife, or mother of a man classified as an enemy, is never considered an enemy. Instead, she and her children are immediately adopted into the conquering *gosa*, and she is made a legitimate member of the community with full rights and responsibilities.

In the rare instance that a woman commits murder, it is her *gosa* that must pay *guma*. If a woman is harmed, her community intervenes on her behalf and punishes the attacker. In this sense, the protection of women's bodies falls in the hands of her blood relations and her husband's clan. Yet, men who have been harmed are encouraged to retaliate on their own. For this reason, a local proverb states that it is through the protection of women's bodies that wars are started; not through the quarreling of men.

Today, the Ethiopian court system administers legal ruling on murder cases and with *guma* outlawed, *heera* can no longer be enforced in the same way. Islamic Shari'a law handles minor offenses and oversees domestic affairs, and, as a result, women's rights have shifted, and their physical value and protection have largely deteriorated. Yet men and women of all ages are aware of *heera* and often recall the exact punishment for death or dismemberment among the various clans in eastern

Oromia. In 2000, I filmed a *guma* reenactment in a remote community in Eastern Hararghe. The male and female actors who participated followed "proper" *guma* action, slaughtering a bull, singing, reciting prayers, interviewing witnesses, and negotiating the blood price. Just as *guma* once allowed elders from the killer's clan to meet with elders from the victim's clan to settle their disputes and agree on a fair price for misconduct or murder, elders today report that such informal meetings are still held, though payment is symbolic and usually not enforceable.

Although *guma* was already banned during the time of the Egyptian Occupation, traditional law is still practiced in rural areas where modern criminal law is not easily accessible or, if jails are full and administrators busy, the national court will allow local laws to be enforced. Even if a man is jailed for a crime by the national courts or the case is settled in Shari'a court, his *gosa* may still demand traditional compensation of 25 cows based on *heera*.

One informant described the outlawing of *heera* with the introduction of Islam:

> In Oromo *heera* every woman or man has the right to be compensated. However, in Islam a woman can't rule or be Imam or be a judge and with Muslim religion, the *guma* is not equal. A woman's death is now half the worth of a man. Then, after Menelik's occupation, all Afran Qallo *heera* was brought underground. There, men discussed what should be done. How would we live with these people [Amharic speakers]? If a man says "*ishī*" [yes, Amharic], he can live. So, we will say "*ishi*," and keep our culture underground. Before the women had formal training in *heera*; today they don't know it since it went underground. (I.A. February 20, 2000)

This passage reflects the current challenges that Muslim Barentuma women face around the protection of their bodies between Oromo traditional laws that protected their mothers and modern Shari'a law. In the first instance, the highest regard is given to the Oromo bodily ideal, a fertile female body, intact and unblemished. In the second case, Islamic mandate dictates a lesser worth for the life of a woman, and further prescribes that her body be hidden because it produces lust in men and seduces harmful *jinn* (supernatural forces). Today, the female body has the potential, essentially, to be too beautiful. Being overly attractive is also cause for concern, since it leaves women vulnerable to the attacks of those with the *buda* (evil eye). This push and pull between Oromo *heera* and Shari'a law is played out through women's complex negotiation of revealing and concealing – not to become too beautiful and a magnet for spirits, jealousy, and reprimand from the mosque or too powerful, like the ruler Mote Qorqee.

Female Bodies and Power: The Legend of Mote Qorqee

Mote Qorqee serves as a regional trope that relates to men's attitudes toward controlling aggressive women. She is described in tales as a cunning and merciless ruler, not unlike the biblical Judith with whom she is often compared. Among

Highland Orthodox Christians in Ethiopia, Judith is the infamous, blood-thirsty ruler who destroyed holy sites during the sixteenth century, and who was finally outsmarted.

The legend of Mote Qorqee is told throughout Oromia regions. *Mote* means "winner" and *qorqee* denotes an antelope or hartebeest. Mote Qorqee is literally the queen of the hartebeest and her stories describe a shrewd, selfish leader. She is called 'Akko Manoyyee' ('Grandmother of Home') among Oromo groups such as the Ittu, Guji, Wollega, and Karreyu, and 'Akko Banoye' among the Oromo-speaking Gabra in Kenya (Wood 1999, 6).

While the feats of her reign are mythic in proportion, some informants have suggested that Mote Qorqee was Queen Yodit Gudit of the south who destroyed Axum or Queen Maya Lama, a celebrated female ruler in the early dynasty of the Harari emirate. Tadiyan Maya Lama reigned twenty-two years after her father Maya, a Muslim emir. She was Afran Qallo, born in Maya Gudoo, located near Haromaya. Maya Lama led her people to Islam, held a large army, established a modern form of government, extended trade relations throughout Oromia and Arabia, and brought rain when there was a drought with the help of Oromo diviners.[42] In contrast to Mote Qorqee, Maya Lama, is considered a just leader who ruled for only a short period.[43]

In any case, the saga of Mote Qorqee is that of an Oromo female ruler from the Alla clan who was born at Qorqee near Haromaya, and who tried to extend her reign throughout the Horn of Africa and beyond to Jiddah, Zeila, and Aden on the southeastern Arabian coast. Since she was only a local ruler of Oromo pastoralists in and near Harar, with no standing army or neighboring allegiances, her aspiration went unrealized. Her reputation as a cruel ruler governed by her desire for power and control extended far and wide through stories of her exploits.

On one occasion, retold by several informants, Mote Qorqee climbed onto a *mooraa* (communal cattle corral) and sat with her legs dangling over the side. She demanded that the cows be let out of the gate without grazing her legs. The frustrated herders went to a nearby cave to see a holy man named 'Biiqqee', to ask for his advice. Caves today are considered powerful spaces inhabited by *jinn* spirits who are attracted to underground springs. While diviners and mystics may take up residence or receive patients in caverns, most people avoid them in daily travels. In the story, Biiqqee happened to be the oldest surviving mystic of the clan because Mote Qorqee, threatened by the power of male elders, had most of them put to death. Biiqqee told the herders to take dried mats of leather and fan the cattle as they moved through the gate. The men followed his advice and in so doing, the cows became frightened by the movement and jumped over Mote Qorqee. Realizing that she had been tricked and that some wise man was surely behind it, she made a second demand. She asked that the *heddii* (small yellow fruit) be loaded onto a camel and transported without the help of rope or bags. Again, the people went to Biiqqee. He told them to take the camel to a muddy place, smear its back with the clay and stick the *heddii* onto its body. When Mote Qorqee saw this, she ordered the entire clan to assemble so that she could seek out the old man who undermined her authority and have him killed. The small Biiqee hid himself in a sack on the back of a young, untrained camel. When Mote Qorqee began her scrutiny of the villagers and their livestock, she overlooked this young camel in her examination.

The people then prepared a *wadaajaa* (prayer ceremony) to ask for the help of Waqaa. *Wadaajaa* refers to a religious ceremony accompanied by *marqaa* (porridge) and *hodja* (drink), the chewing of *khat,* and the singing of religious songs. An assembled group will commonly pray to promote fertility for women and livestock, and to end war, famine, domestic disputes, and illness.[44] During this *wadaajaa,* women drummed, and Mote Qoorqee became ecstatic and ordered the people to bring a hartebeest for her to ride. The old man advised the men to catch a very wild, young antelope and to tie Mote Qorqee's limbs firmly to it. When Mote Qorqee mounted the animal, it began to buck frantically and set off on a stampede throughout the land. Her body parts were subsequently severed along the road from Harar to Jarso. As the story goes: At Bishaan Dacha'oo, Mote Qorqee's legs fell off. At Harmallaa (*harma* is the Oromo word for "breast"; *harmalla* is the name of a post-menopausal woman) her breast was severed and dropped to the ground. At Ija Ginnaa (also referred to as 'Guftalubuc') she lost her *gufta* (hairnet).

The division of the body of Mote Qorqee parallels another fable about the division of a cow during ritual feasting. During her reign, Mote Qorqee divided up meat according to the values she placed on gender and age, and these divisions are still recognized during the sacrifice of a cow during *wadaajaa* and *guma*. The stomach, liver, kidney, and intestine are for post-menopausal women. This fatty part of the cow is the part that Mote Qorqee preferred. The lower back is for girls. Ribs are for boys at puberty. The lump of fat on the lower back near the tail is given to young men in their twenties. Flanks from the sides are for religious leaders. The loin is intended for young women with only one child. Old men consume the breast meat. This division of meat for consumption based on gender and age is practiced among all pastoralists or communities of pastoral extraction in East and Northeast Africa. However, explanations for these divisions vary greatly from those of the Afran Qallo.

This story of Mote Qorqee parallels other tales found throughout Africa that illustrate how women who once commanded power lost their traditional political authority to men (Bamberger 1992). Wood (1999, 7) describes a very similar story told by the Oromo-speaking Gabra in northern Kenya. A female leader called 'Banoye' who demanded impossible feats was ultimately rendered powerless through the actions of men who follow the advice of an orphaned boy. When asked to interpret the antics of Mote Qorqee in the story, Oromo men undoubtedly say that it illustrates, on one level, that women are not well suited for positions of political power and it reinforces Islamic principles that state that only men should hold public office. Yet it is also perceived by men and women as an inherently Oromo tale that suggests the life and values of a previous time. During that time, roughly translated as the era before deep penetration of Islam, women could govern, women could oversee the distribution of meat, and women's actions were remembered in place names and sacrifices.

While it can be argued that some Oromo, especially those groups living near the trade routes, were already identifying themselves as Muslim and practicing Shari'a law at the beginning of or even prior to their arrival in Harar, for centuries this newfound faith existed in tandem with Oromo *heera*. Islamic preaching that came through Muslim merchants via the trading channels with the Red Sea was taken up with zeal by the inhabitants of the walled city. However, not all groups embraced Islam as Harar's urban population had. Neighboring Oromo agriculturalists and semi-nomadic pastoralists did not receive the same exposure to Qur'anic education, and many were only nominally Muslim until the forced conversions implemented during the short-lived Egyptian colonial period (1875–1885). Only a few Nole and Alla Oromo had received much exposure to Islam and Shari'a law, while the Baabile and mixed Somali groups had largely been converted before the Egyptians arrived (M.S.S., March 3, 2000). An Alla Oromo elder recounted his grandfather's story about the days prior to forced conversion at the hands of the Egyptians for those who, like most, still maintained many aspects of their traditional governing system. He states:

> The Arabs came to us three times before the Turks. They came with their book and they took our land. When we learned to read the Qur'an, we recognized some of its principles. It told us: "One man should not touch another man's wives." We realized that this was part of our *seera* [law]. Another law stated: "Don't rob another man's wealth." The Oromo agreed that this, too, was something we understood. The book also told us: "Don't harm peaceful people," and we had accepted this too, a long time ago. We were told by the book to "reap the products of our work" and this we understood. My ancestors thought that they were being tricked and replied: "His is already our law. We knew it before. You conquering Arabs are using this book as your shield." These forefathers killed the Arabs on their first trip and refused them on their second. Then the Arabs researched the Oromo religion and found that we often pray and hold ceremonies for *ayyaana* and Waqaa. They sent *awaliyas* (Islamic spiritual propagandists) to sit with us in our *hujuba*, our cemetery. These *awaliyas* were very organized politically and they settled in many places. When they died, the Muslims made tombs for them. Our forefathers began bringing their dead there and praying: "If this Shaykh is going to heaven, let our dead go with him." (M.S.S., February 27, 2000)

In this statement, we glean the surface similarities between the two faiths. Islamic proselytizers found ways to utilize these similarities to make significant headway in converting the local populations. However, conversion also limited the authority of the Oromo constitution and the vast rights that governed the protection of women and their bodies. After learning of the many protections afforded women in *heera*, I inquired why the beating of women (wives, girlfriends, daughters) by men was now commonplace or at least talked about as an act that went unpenalized. Men and women inevitably responded that the elders who oversaw *heera* were today no longer able to endorse and enforce its laws due to the encroachment of larger

Islamic and state-controlled polices. Further, the time has passed since women, such as Mote Qorqee, could hold office and assert political power.

Siiqee: Women's Scepter of Power

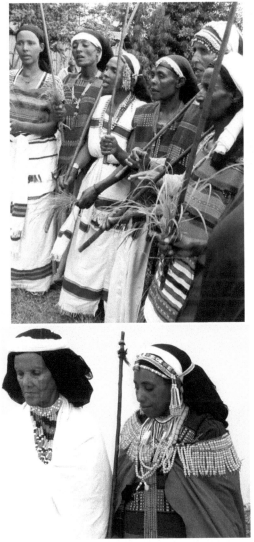

Figure 4.1 Arsi Women holding Siiqee

Yet, there are women's social and religious groups today that wield communal authority, particularly when a woman's rights have been violated. For example, in the spirit possession groups in Harar (discussed in detail in Chapter Five) women under the direction of a spirit can take on temporary leadership roles and men must oblige their demands for compensation for wrongdoing during the ceremony.

Women's prayer groups in Wallo can instigate change by praying and chanting their grievances under a public tree for men to hear. The collective support system known as 'siiqee,' however, is single-handedly the most fundamental advocacy for women's rights.[45] The practice, alive and well in Arsi, has no longer been observed in many other Barentuma areas since the advent of Shari'a law. In its most tangible form, *siiqee* (*sinqee*) is a stick given to women of marriageable age (Figure 4.1). In Wallo, women were given two: one in the shape of 'Y' used for reconciliation, and a straight, unsegmented stick given to her during her wedding. The straight stick is kept throughout her life and goes with a woman to her grave. Men are not allowed to touch it. It functions as a kind of insurance against the potential of unforeseen harm in her marriage. If her husband violates her through physical abuse, verbal harassment, neglect or sexual rejection, a wife may use her stick to summon her female neighbors to her aid. As she steps outside to ululate, wives within earshot are under obligation to cease their pastime, take up their sticks, gather grasses, and follow the caller to a shade tree in the village (Figure 4.2). They will sing: "Our beloved daughter has been dishonored, we will help" (W.B., April 17, 2010).

Women will wait under the tree until the council of men who settle disputes arrives to hear their case. The elders then summon the responsible husband and order him to apologize by slaughtering a sheep or cow and offering his wife and her supporters the meat. Among the Arsi, for example, a woman who has given birth wears *qanafa*, a barrel-shaped forehead ornament that signifies her sacred status for up to five months for a girl child and six months for a boy (Figure 4.3). Her husband may not insult, beat or demand sex from her during this period. If he does, the wife may summon her *siiqee* sisters and demand an apology. If the husband refuses to kill and cook an animal for his wife, the women will curse him, singing: "You, son who is cursed by God, are doing harm. You, oxen who has escaped to Mararow, your name has been spoiled for beating your wife" (W.B., April 17, 2010). If, however, a neighboring woman does not go to the aid of the one wearing *qanafa*, the *siiqee* women may go to her home, take small items, and curse her with the words: "By not coming out of your house to help, we expel you" (G.F., April 17, 2010). In the *siiqee* sisterhood, women are required to go to another women's aid.

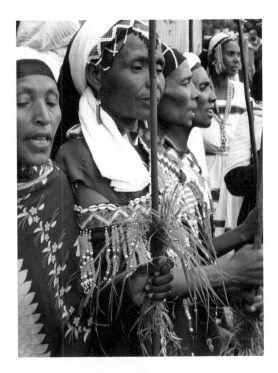

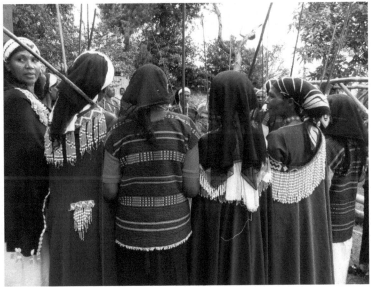

Figure 4.2 Siiqee Women's Group singing

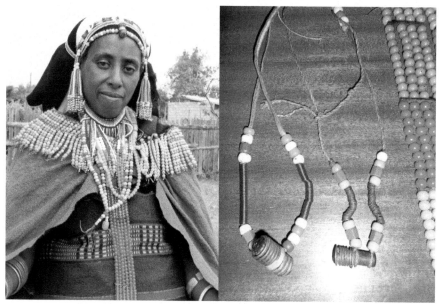

Figure 4.3 The Qanafa, a Barrel-Shaped Forehead Ornament

To sanction the reconciliation between husband and wife, and to honor the stick used to bring women together, the women tie a bit of the sacrificed animal's skin to the top of their stick. A stick covered with many such leather tassels indicates the strength of a woman's support network, her success in reconciling disputes, and her knowledge of *heera* and her rights. Such a woman would be granted a great deal of respect. When she participates in women's prayer ceremonies, women's dance groups or other women-centered gatherings, she will bring with her her *siiqee*. Otherwise, the staff will be kept in the corner of her home, ready to be picked up at a moment's notice if another woman should need her help. In this way, *siiqee* provided women with a means to act if *seera* (laws) had been broken and to restore *saffuu* (peace and sacrality) in the community (Kumsa 1997, 123). Women who have married into Afran Qallo lineages where the *siiqee* institution is not practiced expressed sadness that they no longer had their sticks to protect them. However, within the Oromo Diaspora in the last few years, *siiqee* has become a model for a pan-Oromo women's movement that parallels the male-centered *gada* paradigm as a means of unifying diverse factions in contemporary Oromo politics around the common Oromo ideals of democracy and egalitarianism.

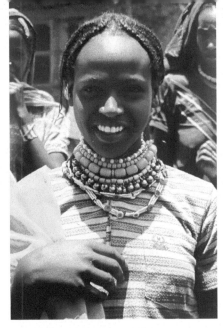

Chapter Five:

Dressing the Spirit/Shielding the Gaze

mina, a beautiful, Oromo woman in her late teens, spends most afternoons in the marketplace selling leafy bundles of *khat*. She sits among a group of Muslim women *khat* sellers, dually companions and competitors, who make their living on the growing past-time of afternoon *khat* chewing among a mostly male clientele. Amina is considered extremely attractive. Her appeal is three-fold: (1) she is physically striking and layers of colorful skirts, bands of seed beads, and tattooed dots on her cheeks further enhance her graces; (2) she is financially secure, spending what money she does not earn for her family on jewelry, cloth, and perfume; and (3) she exhibits a reserved character in accordance with her Islamic upbringing. However, Amina also wears scars between her eyes, shiny metal buttons sewn onto her collar, and leather amulets around her neck to cool and contain her beauty.

Amina is acutely aware that to attract attention is in itself a force that must be closely guarded and kept in check. Young Oromo women have the paradoxical responsibility to attract potential suitors through their physical appeal while repelling harm-inflicting supernatural forces, such as *jinn*, and envious humans with the evil eye called *buda* or *nyaadhu* (those that "eat" with their eyes). Young women are thought to be more susceptible to the attention of *buda* since their youth and use of cosmetics render them too beautiful and potentially causing jealous feelings to surface in others. They are also vulnerable to spirits such as *jarrii*, whom women can gain control over and, on occasion, be possessed by, and quasi-spiritual, totemic animals such as hyenas and snakes. The nature of these dangers requires women to take certain precautions with their bodies, and seek out ritual acts that offer blessings and sacrifice, solicit protection, and implore human and superhuman support.

Adorning the body to beautify, to protect, and/or to welcome a foreign spiritual presence is a complex negotiation. The killing of over 400 Oromo civilians by Ethiopian security forces between November 2015 and June 2017,[46] ongoing drought, and the escalation of the Acquired Immune Deficiency Syndrome (AIDS) epidemic which, to some degree, are all manifested in their effect on the body, further complicate the ways in which Oromo think about the body and, in turn, choose to present it. These contemporary events, as well as particular events in the remembered past, present a deepening need to make sense of death, disease, deformity, and disappearance. Spirit-related performances and supernatural beliefs are one way through which these experiences are elucidated, both tangibly and metaphorically. This chapter moves forward from the previous discussion of identity formation through historical dress to a closer look at the spiritual forces that are captivated by or captivate women: first, through a discussion of body art used as protection against harm (amulets, tattooing, scarring) and the artists that make them, and then through a discussion of body art used in spirit possession. The discussion of the cult of affliction known as '*jarrii*' is framed by a limited set of body art, namely textiles, coins, and feathers, and the ritual accoutrements of the smoking gourd and whip as extensions of bodily dress. This adornment set illustrates the precarious relationships that Amina and others like her engage in during the practice of dress, which includes a desire to make the body attractive and visibly present, while repudiating attention by disguising it. Key in the protection of the body from harm, the containing in the body of benevolent spiritual power, and the ushering forth from the body of grace and beauty are several acts performed by, or onto, the body, including spitting, scarring, shaking, smoking, eating, and hiding. These acts, often associated with rituals of prayer and possession, may require the active expulsion of bodily fluid and body movement or a passive reception to particular acts. These polarized processes further illustrate Oromo notions of the passive and active body as women stay within or stray from prescribed normative behavior.

Oromo bodily extensions, ideals, and acts that herein serve as springboards from which to explore Oromo beliefs about the body, the supernatural, and the environment are never static in meaning. Instead, their meanings fluctuate through time and circumstance; for example, Oromo women may use a large *foota* (scarf) to cover their hair in a public display of modesty, while swinging the corner to coyly flirt with certain passersby. Shiny metal cylindrical amulets and stitched leather pouches threaded on twine filled with Qur'anic formulas are designed both to identify a woman as Muslim to a local audience, while arresting supernatural powers that are believed to be transferred through the gaze. Further, many of the ornaments and objects that figure prominently in historical identity and lifecycle rituals, can and do hold meaning on a metaphysical level as well. One practical reason for this recycling of existing dress within different contextual arenas is the fact that Oromo women, particularly those who reside in the countryside, may only be able to afford a limited repertoire of costumes and accessories. Yet, these types of body art have histories themselves and do not function merely as blank slates on which new meaning is assigned. Rather, their meanings and potencies gather and shift throughout the life of the object and in each new context that they appear.

Shielding the Gaze: *Qarxasaa*

Amina is not alone in the wearing of amulets. Almost all ethnic groups and age groups in Ethiopia wear cases made of leather, paper or metal called '*qarxasaa*' or '*qudhaama*' ('*hirtz*' in Arabic) by the Oromo to guard against such diverse things as bullets, madness, headaches, enemies, wild animals, and harmful spirits. Most *qarxasaa* are sewn leather pouches made by Muslim sheiks in which Arabic or Oromo passages from the Qur'an or horoscope texts are written on pieces of paper or sheepskin and inserted (Figure 5.1). Both Christians and Muslims wear amulets predominantly to ward off *buda*. Like the leather miniatures prepared with herbs and incantations by Orthodox Christian *debtera* (low-class priests) it is the power of the holy written word encased in leather that protects the wearer. In the Christian case, *debteras* combine biblical images with gospel passages and the names of God in order "to assure the salvation of the one who writes it, reads it, explains it, buys it, and wears it, up to the seventh generation" (Mercier 1979, 13). In the case of an ongoing illness, a *debtera* utilizes painted scrolls to help drive out local spirits, known collectively as '*zar*' or to placate them within the host and protect the host from further encounters. In lieu of painted parchment with Christian imagery, Muslim amulets might include graphic patterns from the Oromo horoscope texts.

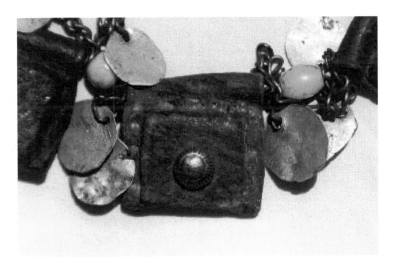

Figure 5.1 Qarxasaa with Metal Inlay strung with Metal Disks and Beads

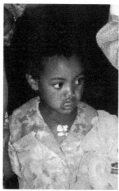

Figure 5.2 Young Oromo Girl wearing Paper Amulet

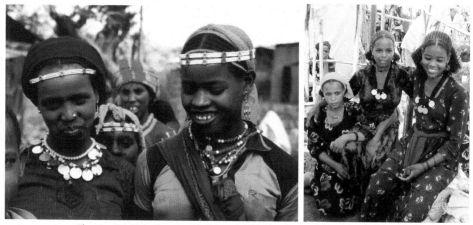

Figure 5.3 Girls from Baabile and Wallo wearing Coin Amulets

Baabile Oromo who live east of Harar claim that the Amharic term 'buda' (which can refer to an artisan caste, the individual with the evil eye or the act of inflicting harm through the gaze) was not familiar to the Oromo until the introduction of Harar into the Ethiopian Empire under Emperors Menelik and Haile Selassie. As one male informant stated:

> Buda came with Christianity, Amhara, and the feudal system. We Oromo did not have this concept of evil. The Amhara have a real fear of concentrated power. The Oromo do not fear this power. In fact, we use it to our advantage when we pray together during wadaajaa. Buda is the person with the evil eye who does harm to others by bringing illness when he or she feels jealousy or anger. It can only be cured through the use of qumbii (incense), the reading of the Qur'an, or intense beatings. We too take precautions to ward off buda since they [buda] are now among us and we have adopted their [Amhara] ways. (A.M., April 6, 2000)

While the reading of the Qur'an, the burning of incense, and severe beatings can drive inherent evil from the person with buda, those particularly susceptible to attacks by the evil eye, namely young women, will also don leather amulets, coins, and scars as visual protection from the *buda*'s gaze. If a *buda* does strike, the behavior of the afflicted (including shaking, shouting, and speaking in a foreign tongue) mimics possession by a spirit. While *buda* is conceived of as a foreign presence that was introduced under the feudal system during Abyssinian rule, it is in the realm of experience of both Qur'anic *jinn* spirits and Oromo *jarrii* spirits who each may manifest as possessing forces. In each case, leather amulets function as spiritual repellents or talismanic signifiers.

While the holiest part of the amulet for both Muslims and Christians – the sacred wrapped text – is hidden from view, to be efficacious, the amulet must be visible to the person with the evil eye. Young Oromo women most commonly decorate their upper chests and throats with strung amulets, since this is often the focal point for the eye when two people first encounter one another. The three most common types of amulets worn by the Barentuma Oromo include paper squares, leather pouches filled with Qur'anic verses, and items that glisten in the sun (Figures 5.1, 5.2, 5.3). To draw attention to the amulet and its hidden, protective power and away from the wearer's eye, shiny metal beads, coins or buttons are added to the body to catch sunlight and charm the eye away from the face. Once the eye of the *buda* is directed toward a leather or metal amulet, his or her intrinsic destructive power is harnessed either in the amuletic pocket or immediately reflected by the coin. In a similar fashion, Moroccan Amazigh women weave "eye-catching motifs" into their textiles to harness the evil eye (Becker 2006b, 44). Once harnessed or reflected, the *buda* and the wearer can safely look each other in the eye without adverse side-effects. Paulitschke (1896, 31) reports that when Oromo and Somali were first exposed to the gleaming metal of foreign gun barrels and the awesome power to transform life to death in the guns themselves, shiny substances became the most potent ornaments against death and misfortune. Pieces of metal, amber, and, later, coins, become important talismans in their own right, and are seen today worn alone or with leather *qarxasaa*. It should be mentioned that the neighboring Argobba have recreated the look of the Oromo leather *qarxasaa* by carving smaller versions in wood that are then strung onto a necklace with beads. Young men carve the small cases in their free time for women to assemble and wear. Argobba women who wore the necklace say that the cases are intended only for beauty and they do not hold the thaumaturgical function that they do for the Oromo because they do not hold the secret text. It is the hidden verse that is efficacious.

From Paulitschke's (1896, 31) observations in the 1880s, we can be sure that Amina's great grandmother was also familiar with the use of leather pouches to hold pieces of Qur'anic script written by specialists worn on the neck and less frequently on the arm. He mentions that historically, amber, teeth, and bird claws were the usual accompaniments with which the leather pouches were strung. The most common amulets of animal extraction today are the skin or liver of the hyena and antelope or dikdik jaws, with the back teeth attached worn on the arm by adults and on the neck by children.

Qarxasaa are often categorized as created for two groups: (1) those intended for children and (2) those for beautiful and/or successful adults. These groups, ripe with potential, are most likely to instill feelings of jealousy in others. Jealously within the Oromo belief system has the ability to manifest as physical harm with or without the conscious intentions of the seer. The emotion arises due to the perception of another's advantages and manifests as attacks to the victim's body. This assault can range from disfigurement to disease. During a smallpox epidemic in the late 1960s, remembered in the town of Kemise in south Wallo, traditional healers are said to have inoculated certain townspeople by rubbing pus from the infected into open wounds of the healthy, all the while blessing the disease through song. In singing the praises and thereby anthropomorphizing the disease, those jealous *buda* thought to be responsible for its initial spread, were placated and their "biting eyes" made impotent. Near the site of the wound, an amulet was tied to ward off further harm. This story illustrates a number of important points that reoccur in discussions of *buda*: (1) jealously can cause illness, (2) illness is physically connected to the attacker, (3), placating the illness, and, in turn, the attacker can leave the affliction impotent, and (4) amulets guard vulnerable places on the body.

Precarious Occupations: *Tumtuu, Waata* and *Ogeesa*

The concept of the evil eye is situated in Christian and Muslim communities throughout the Horn of Africa, and rooted, to a lesser extent, in early civilizations in North Africa and the Middle East. The evil eye as a pan-Ethiopian phenomenon is most widely known as '*buda*', a term that designates both the inherent eye power and the individuals who possess it; usually castes that smelt iron, tan leather, and fashion pots as their primary means of livelihood. In Ethiopia, *buda* is most closely associated with an endogamous class of blacksmiths who make tools and weapons, and who historically also produced *qarxasaa* in less Islamized areas. Among the Oromo, those who heat and hammer metal with a forge, and create simple tools are known as '*tumtuu*', a term that also refers to *tumtuu* (tattooing) or the hammering of a green-black paste made of soot and plant extract into the skin with a thorn or needle. In eastern Ethiopia, *tumtuu* were largely applied by endogamous Midigaan Somali men who became the primary suppliers of tools, weapons, and jewelry to the populations near Harar in the early nineteenth century, while their wives worked as potters. *Tumtuu* are classified as unpredictable, polluted, and dangerous by Oromo today, not unlike the characterization of *buda* throughout Ethiopia. The creation of tattoos on the face is believed to mimic the magical practice of smithing practiced by the *tumtuu*. In this regard, by mimicking the hammering motions of the *tumtuu* as he transforms metal, the tattooist transforms the face, granting it a second skin that both draws attention to this region and disguises it. As Gell (1993, 32) states, the tattooed skin becomes a kind of container that presents and withholds information. Tattoos can range from one tiny dot on a cheek to bold, ankh-like shapes between the eyebrows and V-shaped patterns around the mouth and cheeks. Tattooing the face with blue ink along the bridge of the nose, the eyebrows, around the eyes, and on the neck has been practiced in Oromia for at least six generations (Paulitschke 1888a, 69).

By the mid-nineteenth century, "an outcast, but tolerated" group of blacksmiths who were believed to have the evil eye were living in the countryside surrounding the walled city of Harar (Caulk 1977, 374). Later, the southern gate of Harar became known as '*buda* gate' since the neighborhood beyond this gate was inhabited by metalworking families, who, due to their occupation, were regarded as tainted with the evil eye. Like the Jewish Falasha potters who are situated near Gondar in northwestern Ethiopia, *tumtuu* are despised because they usually do not own land, work the land as farmers or participate in animal husbandry. Further, they are thought to have the capacity to become hyenas and devour unsuspecting villagers who venture out at night. Yet, it is the *tumtuu* that historically fashioned the *qarxasaa*. And the sheiks who are today responsible for their creation, utilize hyena leather for their most potent creations. Like the smallpox incident discussed above, the Oromo become spiritually strong by harnessing that which is spiritually dangerous. In the case of the *tumtuu*, it is he who makes the object that will protect others from him. In the case of the hyena, the sheik uses the skin of the hyena to guard against hyena attacks.

Oromo informants mention that prior to the arrival of Muslim foreigners and the arrival of *tumtuu*, Oromo had trade relations with *waata*, a tribe of male hunters, female gatherers, and male and female craftspeople who produced leather, weapons, poisons, and pottery. In Oromo *seera* (indigenous oral law) *waata* were not only in charge of producing all jewelry, tools, shields, and domestic items, they were also in charge of caring for Oromo children and characterized as endowed with spiritual wisdom that was manifest through "eye power" (A.S.J., October 11, 2000). In this case, the eye power of the *waata* was considered a positive attribute that allowed them to be extraordinary hunters and diviners with the ability to "see" game hidden in the forest and "foresee" that which was to occur. Today, most Oromo refer to the semi-nomadic groups of *waata* who once lived in the east as 'munyoo' or '*bon.*' *Munyoo* are thought to have fled Oromia during the invasion of Menelik II and trekked to south central Kenya near Mt. Kilamanjaro, where they no longer hunt, but, instead, help Borana Oromo "on their journey through their ability to speak with crocodiles and birds, bring honey and sap from trees, extract medicines and poisons from plants, and make amulets" (M.S.S., March 3, 2000). Kassam and Bashuna (2004, 198) paint a more desperate picture in which *waata*, who today are no longer able to hunt or gather due to Kenyan national park regulations, live in poverty.

In 1969, Huntingford (1965, 16) described *waata* as a pariah group of hippopotamus hunters found throughout Ethiopia and the Kenyan coast who "live either in subjection to or in some sort of symbiosis with their more advanced neighbors." This would seem to contradict the present Barentuma Oromo conception of *waata* as the great hunters of their past. It is certainly possible that they are not referring to the same groups since as Brooke (1956, 74) clearly points out: "inasmuch as different groups of people known as '*waata*' are found in nearly all parts of Ethiopia, it has been suggested that the word 'waata' is a generic name of a class of ethnically diverse hunting peoples." However, it is also likely that this notion of ambiguity in which *waata* hold both high and low status, depending on the audience, is in conformity with the characterization of other landless, occupational castes who engage in hunting, smithing, or potting throughout Africa as powerful and also dangerous.

The Wallo Oromo call those who made farming tools and jewelry in the past '*ogeesa*.' *Ogeesa* are also responsible for fixing the broken bones and pulled muscles of people and animals. They are highly praised as healers and craftspeople, and command great respect. Unlike *tumtuu*, *waata* and *ogeesa* are considered positions of prestige and honor for most Oromo today. Each of these occupations, nonetheless, are body practitioners who make and utilize objects connected to spiritual protection or who themselves have transformative power. In each case, this spiritual power is associated with the Oromo concept of polarized energy – eye power – which can assist or abuse. In a similar fashion, specific body art, such as scars made by the tattoo artists, are understood to repel and attract simultaneously.

Facial Scarring and Haile Selassie

Scars called '*haaxixa*' (*ibirku*), incised with a sharp thorn or razor that lacerates the first few layers of skin above the eyebrow, along the bridge of the nose, and on the cheeks are usually made at the onset of puberty, and become meaningful on several levels: when those above the eye are cut, the blood is allowed to drip down and cleanse the eyeball, believed to free it from eye disease; the mark along the nose is intended to visually lengthen the nose and enhance its appeal; the marks on the cheeks further beautify a woman's face and suggest regional identity. Often, *haaxixa* are paired with tattooing (*tumtuu*) (Figure 5.4). As a result, the natural appearance of the face is masked through minor disfigurement. While this disfigurement is thought of as cosmetic today which makes women more attractive, it is also meant to divert the gaze of strangers from initial consideration of the eyes. This is the key paradox of Oromo women's body art.

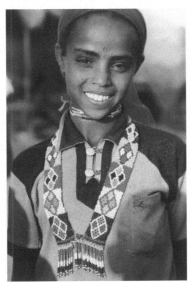

5.4 An Afran Qallo Girl wearing Beaded Ambarka and Scars (Haaxixa) paired with Tattooing (Tumtuu)

Just as *waata* and *ogeesa* are recorded as highly esteemed professions in Oromo traditional law, while *tumtuu* held a more negative association that was later transferred to *buda* when it was introduced during Abyssinian imperial rule, the practice of scarring the face is also reported to have been used in a different way during Haile Selassie's first reign (1930–1941) – in this case, to make ugly, rather than to beautify. The Oromo speak of a tumultuous time in the 1920s when young men and women began disappearing in great numbers. As most Barentuma Oromo groups had had little exposure to Ethiopia's government or state-sponsored education at this period, an uncertainty grew concerning the motivations of a distant leader called 'Haile Selassie.' Severe changes to Oromo land use, the complete eradication of the traditional socio-political governing institutions, and new demands for labor and a national militia created mounting distrust toward the Ethiopian state. Informants state that in the 1930s, it was confirmed by a famous Oromo *mantiyya* (a *jarrii* spirit expert) that Haile Selassie was himself possessed by an Amhara *buda* spirit (A.S.J., February 25, 2000). This spirit was said to inhabit his dog, a Chihuahua breed with bulging eyes, who often appeared with his master in official photographs and news broadcasts. Chihuahuas had not been seen by the majority of Ethiopians before. An Oromo woman recounted that people feared that the small dog was masterfully controlling Haile Selassie to tour the country to collect and consume the most attractive people (M.M., March 5, 2000). As a result, the most beautiful Oromo men and women were being confiscated by government troops and eaten by this insatiable ruler. Mothers began to hide their children and severely scar their faces to keep them from abduction (M.M., March 10, 2000; A.A.J., May 16, 2010). In this sense, excessive *haaxixa* was used as a means of marring beauty and keeping young men and women safe. Oromo in the east claim that the harshness of the Abyssinian administration, especially from 1887 to 1936, and the fear of *buda* that ensued brought about an increase in the wearing of scars, coins, and amulets at this time.

Dressing the Spirit: *Jarrii* Possession

Scholars who have examined possession in Ethiopia (*zar, ayyaana, jinn, setani*) have largely focused on functional explanations concerning the therapeutic value of spirit affliction as either a way of confronting social change (Braukämper 1983; Hinnant 1970, 1990) or as a deprivation cult for marginalized groups to gain access to experiences and forms not readily available to them, including fine clothes, meat, and the roles of foreigners and rulers (Dahl 1989; Hamer 1966; Leiris 1938; I. M Lewis 1989; Messing 1958; Shack 1971). For example, among the Borana, Aguilar (1994, 201) mentions that all female participants, not just the woman possessed, "gain a ritual power which by all current Islamic standards is not supposed to dwell with them." H. Lewis (1982, 471) writes that to classify spirit possession practices in Ethiopia by name and type is itself useless, since spirit possession is a phenomenon "truly protean, exceedingly variable, capable of all manner of elaboration and recombination." After reading these studies and assuming spirit possession would be found among the Eastern Oromo (Azais and Chambard 1931; Morton 1973; Waldron 1974), I was surprised to find informants responding with confused looks when I first began asking about *ayyaana* possession performances in and around Harar in 1998. Ultimately, I learned that Lewis' protean understanding of the practice was correct. It took eight months of inquiry before I realized I had been using the wrong name (they call it '*jarrii*' not '*ayyaana*') and I found Muslim Barentuma women who would admit to practicing it.

The wide-ranging definitions of '*ayyaana*' suggests just how many variables are at play when trying to make sense of a belief system and practice (Hassen 2017, 25). While the concept of *ayyaana* as a possessing spirit is still prevalent among the Borana Oromo, it is absent among most Barentuma Oromo, though the word is still part of their vocabulary – meaning, among other things, a healing essence, fate, luck, personal destiny, a celebratory occasion and more rarely, a collective lineage or guardian spirit.

An early account from the Hararghe region comes from Paulitschke (1896, 22) who classifies *ayyaana* as a guardian angel. He says that to the unlucky was often said "*ajanike sin djaladu*," meaning, "your guardian spirit does not love you." Elderly informants also remembered this more antiquated association of *ayyaana* as guardian spirits to whom the Oromo once prayed (S.M.G., April 4, 2000). One informant mentioned that the Baabile still called *ayyaana* a lineage ancestor when sickness befell them, but most would never admit to using it (M.A.H., March 14, 2000). In the past, the great *ayyaana* of Barentuma could also be called by name to ensure peace as could the *ayyaana* of Sheik Hussein in Bale whose tomb is the most holy pilgrimage site for Muslim Oromo.

Those informants who talked of *ayyaana* as a kind of fate mentioned that *ayyaana* was never in conflict with a person's own will before Islam or Christianity had penetrated Oromo lands (A.S.J., February 9, 2000). It is said that with the coming of both religions, *setani* (demons) began to interfere with people's minds and caused the *ayyaana* to quarrel. In addition, the sacrifices and prayers that were once reserved for the *ayyaana* of lineages and nature were, instead, placed before Muslim *awaliyas* (saints) at tomb sites. Innumerable shrines devoted to heroes, rulers, and individuals who have performed miracles can be found throughout Harar and the surrounding area (Gibb 1996, 1998, 1999; Waldron 1974). As one Afran Qallo woman noted: "People who are Muslim converts would pray to *ayyaana*, and then return to their foreign religion. The *ayyaana* arrested them and they became crazy" (K.A.M., April 12, 2000). Some describe this transfer of devotion from *ayyaana* to *awaliya* as a kind of early propaganda brought by Muslim proselytizers. One accounts states:

> *Ayyaana* is the power that *Waqaa* sent down to earth to watch over people and help them. When we are caught by drought or stricken by disease and catastrophe, we used to pray to Waqaa. In Islam, similarly, we may worship Allah through the *awaliyas*. When the first Muslim missionaries came here, they carried with them the power of the *awaliyas*. They told the Oromo the story of how Abadir and the forty-four *awaliyas* rode into town on lions and elephants. They convinced the Oromo that these *awaliya* were *ayyaana*, spirits that would live on forever and help them. After the Oromo left *raba-dori* and other traditional practices, the remaining great *ayyaana* spirits went into hiding in the forest. Those *ayyaana* that agreed with Muslim and Christian spirits stayed on. Now these *ayyaana* speak only non-Oromo languages and may lash out at us. (A.S.I., February 25, 2000)

Perhaps, therefore, the use of the term '*ayyaana*', which once signified a positive essence but today is less understood, has fallen into disuse as a spiritual power.

Ayyaana is also part of the traditional Barentuma Oromo horoscope calendar based on celestial movements. The practice of consulting the horoscope to understand one's natural inclination and as a guideline for one's life course is found almost exclusively today among the Karrayyu and Arsi Oromo. Each month is divided into twenty-seven days, and each day has its own *ayyaana* and name. For example, if a baby is born on Innikah (the first day of the month), this child will take on the disposition and destiny associated with this day, and exemplify the character and power of that *ayyaana*.

Today, *ayyaana* is no longer thought of as a specific spirit, but as a positive, secularized philosophical condition that relates to ritual activities associated with the blessing of humans, nature, and lineage ancestors. Among the Christian Ittu Oromo, for example, the collective Christian saints are called '*ayyaana*.' Among them, the Marii (Virgin Mary) is the most common *ayyaana* spirit invoked in prayer, particularly during women's *atete* ceremonies.[47] For the Arsi, *ayyaana* is intimately connected to the Oromo traditional supreme being Waqaa. Bartels (1975, 889) states that "*ayyanna* is Waqaa in a special way; it is Waqaa in relation to particular events, persons and groups; it is Waqaa's creative power in a person, an animal, a plant, a clan or an animal species as a whole, making them the way they are." In general, the *ayyaana* that exists in each human being is generally described as a positive force that determines and guides one's life path. While one would not pray to one's own *ayyaana*, more powerful *ayyaana* could be consulted in prayer and summoned during sacrifice. The elders are thought to possess powerful *ayyaana*, which family members elicit through the blessings of *tufta* (aspersion), sprayed onto the forehead and hair.[48]

Jinn

Nowadays, many Barentuma Oromo identify themselves as Muslim and most have had some formal Islamic schooling. Male and female students learn entire passages of the Qur'an by heart in madrasas. In the Qur'an, *jinn* (and *setani*) are mentioned over two dozen times and an entire Surat al-Jinn is devoted to the topic. Although *jinn* (*jnoun* in North Africa) are acknowledged in the Qur'an as spirits of fire with the potential for good or evil, Oromo informants state that they believed in their existence long before Islam proselytizers came to the region. The origins of Islamic *jinn* along with *jarrii* and *zar* are explained in the following popular narrative:

> One day, during the time of Solomon, Allah sent down angels to count how many children Hawa (Eve) had. Fearing that the angels would take her children, Hawa hid the most beautiful children in a cave and displayed only the ugly ones. But Allah knew what Hawa had done and decided to punish her. He turned her beautiful children into *jarrii*. These *jarrii* then wanted to marry one another. But there were not enough sisters to go around, so Adam built a golden house in Gondar for the remaining unwed brothers, Mammaa and Warar. They became the fathers of *zar* and *jinn*, the spirit possession practiced throughout northwestern Ethiopia and the Sudan. At this time Solomon himself controlled all spirits but Mammaa and Warar broke free from his control.
>
> The brothers still live in this golden palace in Gondar but only to those who devote themselves completely to the brothers, make themselves visible. The Oromo families that still worship Mammaa and Warar are Warra Khadanaan Khuudduun, Warra Shauqaar, Maaram Yuuyyoo, and Warra Xuqaar. When Nole Oromo perform *jarrii* ceremonies, they mention Mammaa and Warar as the elders of *jarrii*.[49] (K.A.M., April 12, 2000)

In this story, the most beautiful of Eve's children become *jarrii* and create the spirits *zar* and *jinn*. These forces became somewhat interchangeable in my discussions with informants as they stem from the same essence and each is kept at bay today through daily readings of the Qur'an, using incense, smoking, and praying when entering foreign spaces, enclosed areas, dirty places, and springs.

The underground spring that emerges at the base of a mountain near the village of Ganda Bobeeii near Fedis is renowned for the many *jinn* that inhabit it. A local story recounts that in the early morning, villagers on a fishing expedition or on their way to the market encountered many *jinn* sitting near the spring. People feared them greatly and avoided the area whenever possible. One day, an educated sheik who knew the entire Qur'an by heart, learned of the people's apprehension and went inside a cave near the spring to speak with the *jinn*. They held meetings together for thirteen days. The sheik found that the *jinn* were living like the Oromo – they had a thriving market, a standing army, and a great deal of wealth.[50] When the sheik questioned the *jinn* about where they had come from, they told him that they were children of Allah. The sheik explained that the people were fearful of the *jinn* and therefore avoided the spring. The *jinn* could not understand why people were afraid. For years, the *jinn* had been leaving small gifts of gold near the spring for the Oromo community. The sheik replied that people were ignorant and illiterate, and could not read the Qur'an. The *jinn* explained that they meant the people no harm and that they would, from that point forward, hide when humans passed by or came to fetch water.

In this tale, the sheik ends by telling the *jinn* that if the people only knew the Qur'an, they would be free of their fears. They would know the good *jinn* from the bad, and they would pray and burn incense to keep the bad *jinn* away. Incense is an important ingredient in almost any social occasion throughout Ethiopia but in the recognition of both *jinn* and *jarrii,* it is essential for its potent sweet aroma and the smoke that carries it. Incense is described as air that has been contained. Unlike wind, which is not only characterized as unruly and destructive, but as the culprit to a series of sicknesses, incense drives negative forces away that detest the sweet fragrance. Illnesses that affect the chest, such as pneumonia or tuberculosis are said to be caused by the bad *jinn* manifest as wind. The only protection is to wrap oneself in jackets and scarves, and keep vehicle windows tightly closed so that no skin is exposed to the wind. If an individual is caught uncovered in a gust of wind, she may fall prey to physical deformity, particularly the conditions of leprosy and the turning of the skin to white and dry. In northern Sudan, *zaryan*, or possessing *jinn* associated with the color red, are also referred to as 'red winds' (Boddy 1989, 164, 187). Both conditions threaten smooth, shiny skin – a woman's model state of beauty. Depending on the strength of the *jinn* and the degree of its anger, these conditions can range from temporary and mild to severe and permanent.

Negative *jinn,* recognized as beings of fire created by Allah, are thought to travel with the wind and therefore the wind is always regarded as potentially harmful. Incense, however, is wind rendered harmless; a slow, steady and controlled stream of smoke that placates and pleases positive *jinn,* and cooperative *jarrii* as it rises to the sky. During the pan-Ethiopian coffee ceremony, which may take place three or more times each day, smoke from rock incense contained in white ceramic bowls is waved in front of all present, and most participants never miss a chance to cup and sweep handfuls of the smoke over their foreheads. Further, the woman of the house will bring out bottles of perfume and anoint several times over, the neck and chest of all present. This is thought also to lure away any unwanted *jinn* through the controlled spray of a sweet smell. The importance of smoke in ceremonies extends back at least to the mid-1800s. Burton (1987, 140) reports that tree gum "is thrown upon the fire, and the women are in the habit of standing over it." In Wallo today, most compounds have a shallow pit intended for women's *qayyaa* (smoke baths). Women squat over sweet-smelling, smoking wood chips, and then seal themselves vaginally with cloth or leaves to promote physical and spiritual cleansing. Further, there are cases of Wallo women drinking perfume or a glass of water with the *tufta* (spray blessing of saliva) of women in their spiritual group to directly cleanse and protect their body from *jinn*. In other instances, Wallo Oromo women inflicted with *jinn* paint their bodies with the blood of slaughtered sacrificial animals, enticing the spirit to jump from their bodies and devour the meat.

I found that the terms '*jinn*' and '*jarrii*' were at times used interchangeably when describing spirits who reside near Oromo dwellings and who have a positive effect on humans when they are properly honored. However, when pressed, informants usually differentiated their level of authority: *jinn* are the servants of *jarrii*. Today, in the most heavily Islamized areas among the Barentuma Oromo, *jinn* designate possessing spirits exclusively. *Jinn* can plague an individual, and the means of affliction and the ceremony to follow are similarly described as *jarrii* or they can affect an entire village. In Kemise in Wallo, communal *jinn* spirits called '*baaditti*' (female) and '*baadichaa*' (male) are offered porridge, coffee, and, occasionally, meat on Sundays and Thursdays under a large tree. They are thought of as communal spirits who safeguard the environment from natural calamities. The *jinn* that disturb individuals in Kemise are recognized through a *wadaajaa* prayer ceremony. The victim who shouts and speaks in tongues is meant to sit in the house of the *wadaajaa* leader. A container filled with a mixture of ash and coffee residue is hidden outside the house. The victim and her *jinn* must find the container and drink its contents. This signifies that the person is cured and the *wadaajaa* is successful. The *jinn* will leave the patient and she will continue to provide annual sacrifices to him and don the colors, smells, and textures he desires.

Jarrii and the Possession Ritual

Oromo women in Harar state that the belief in *jarrii* spirits, which came to Harar with the advent of Islam, is much older than the belief in *buda*. While *buda* and *jinn* can be redirected with the wearing of a *qarxasaa*, the uttering of Qur'anic verses, *shisha* (smoking a water pipe), and the burning of rock incense, *jarrii* can only be managed through repetitive ceremony and sacrifice.

In ancient times, there was no *jarrii* or *buda* in Harar, only *awaliyas* or Islamic saints, as one story goes. One day a Muslim man named 'Sheik Haashiim,' patron saint of the poor and crazy according to Gibb (1996, 89, 12), who had come to Harar with the Muslim saint Aw Abadir between the tenth and twelfth century, prayed to Allah calling him "Yaa Waduud." When he said this, people in the area joked with him, saying that what he had really uttered was "Yaa Wadooyee," the name for all *jarrii* spirits collectively. Sheik Haashiim denied the people's accusation but the people continued to pester him. When the people refused to leave Haashiim alone, he called over his shoulder to the *jarrii*: "All right, get in." In the following months people who had pestered Hasshiim grew sick, mad, or lame. Since that day, *jarrii* have been able to enter the five gates of the old city and afflict humans (K.A.M., April 12, 2000). The Wallo Oromo, however, state that *jarrii* came more recently and from the Amhara and that the term comes from the Amharic *zar* or *zarrii*, though because there is no 'z' in the Oromo language, is pronounced with a 'j.' In ancient times, long before the time of King Menelik (1865–1889) and the Emperor (1889–1913) when the Amhara and Oromo were fighting, aggressive Oromo warriors captured Amhara women and cattle. These women and cattle had *jarrii*. When Oromo men married the captured women and incorporated the cows into their herds, the *jarrii* jumped on the backs of Oromo people and their animals. The new human hosts were made to jump, shake, shout, and speak Amharic. A line from a song among the Karrayyu states: "Please leave *jarrii*, you non-Oromo or Amhara from the mountain." (In this case, *sidama* or *sidaam* is used to designate 'foreigner').

Regardless of the historical accuracy of when certain beliefs entered the Oromo milieu, the moral message of the tales above reminds people that spirits will only harm those who exhibit bad behavior. Unlike *buda*, which is a human force motivated by jealousy or greed, the *jarrii* spirit preys on individuals who neglect prescribed codes of conduct. Owing to the very nature of attraction as a force that can draw forth harm, beauty is never free from its associations with jealousy and therefore, women practice reserve when giving and receiving compliments on appearances. Victims are unanimously women, since women through their women's associations bear the responsibility of handling non-Islamic spiritual matters for their families and clans. Yet once possessed, women are free to act outside of prescribed norms.

When good behavior coupled with *qarxasaa*, scars, and tattoos fails to keep harmful spirits at bay, a *jarrii* ceremony may be performed. The central objects in *jarrii* ceremonies among the Afran Qallo are imported cloth, Italian coins, decorated gourd pipes, feathers, and whips. This next section examines how these decorations and accoutrements come into play once someone who has been unsuccessful in repelling a *jarrii* spirit is afflicted or possessed by it and seeks out ritual service.

The *Jarrii* Ceremony

Jarrii is but one of many ceremonies enacted by particular Oromo women's religious groups each year, including Challee in June, a ritual for the female spirit Gamura in January, the Muslim ceremony Wasanu in September, and Eid al-Fitr at the end of Ramadan. Most *jarrii* ceremonies take place over eight days, with each day devoted to a different spirit. *Jarrii* spirits in eastern Oromia are classified into twelve clan names modeled after Oromo genealogy, with each clan housing a long line of descendants. When a ceremony is performed, usually all major ancestral spirits are recognized. In this sense, the *jarrii* ceremony reproduces the known social world of the Barentuma Oromo.

Most *jarrii* are male spirits who may sing songs about genealogy and warfare; two realms in which women do not normally participate. Since Oromo women marry outside their clan, they are not expected to recall their father's genealogy, and since warfare is defined within familial categories, they are not expected to remember past battles and the names of fallen heroes. Oromo men, however, may be able to recite the military accomplishments of their direct male ancestors, ten to forty generations removed. Today, among more Islamized Oromo communities where parallel-cousin marriage is actually preferred to exogamous villages composed of patrilineages who have corporate ownership of land and stock, women have better access to family histories, but they are no longer as important to remember. Even though women are not expected to know a great deal about past deeds and family histories, *jarrii* possession reveals significant knowledge about important local heroes and events.

Each *jarrii* spirit has distinct attributes, including unique culinary, color, and adornment desires; for example, the Amhara spirit Addannee requires the staple *injera* (pancake), tobacco, cigarettes, alcohol, the sacrifice of a white sheep, and white clothing. The spirit Baaba Anooroo requires *khat*, tobacco with ash, stuffed intestines, the sacrifice of a red hen, and shiny red and pink clothing. These objects were described as lures used to attract the spirits to the world of the living and become interested in human affairs (M.S., March 27, 2000).

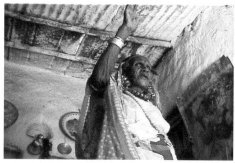 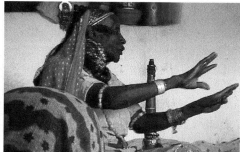

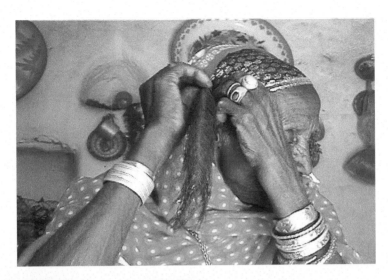

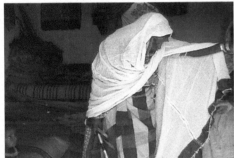 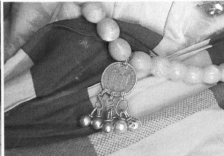

5.5 Aasha prepares for a Jarrii Ceremony with Ostrich Feathers, Coins, Whip, and Cloth

The *mantiyya,* the ritual expert and overseer of the *jarrii* ceremony, is an inherited position held almost exclusively by financially independent, post-menopausal women. Aasha, in her eighties, has been a *mantiyya* for every ethnic group in and around Harar (Oromo, Harari, Somali, Argobba, Afar, Amhara) for over fifty years (Figure 5.5). She wears *baalli guchii* (feather of an ostrich), a colorful tartan wrap, and yellow *challee* (beads) with *chinko* (Italian coins). At her neck is *arwo,* red amber from Mogadishu that she acquired for her *jarrii* during the Italian Occupation (1936–1941) and which she never takes off. She also wears other necklaces and bracelets that are gifts from clients. During a ceremony, Aasha and her client wear the same clothes throughout the performance, unifying them with the common spirit. Aasha's position as *mantiyya* came about after a serious illness as a child and a series of visits by spirits in dreams. This experience parallels the accounts of other *mantiyya.*

Kadija, another *jarrii mantiyya* living within the old city of Harar, was interviewed in her home one afternoon in mid-April 2000. She smoked a large water pipe and chewed *khat,* while a young girl staffed the coals and popped popcorn in the courtyard while we spoke (Figure 5.6). Kadija began describing *jarrii* spirits in only the most nondescript way, for she felt that if she were to utter their names, they would harm her. She began the interview by warning: "I go all places to do *jarrii* for people, but I can't tell you where they came from or their names. If I pronounce their name, they will come now" (K.A.M., April 12, 14, 2000). In fact, she did say their names on a few occasions, but the utterances were followed by handfuls of popcorns tossed to the ground, the spitting of water, and verbal blessings. She said that she could not say the names of spirits unless she gave them the material things that they desired – popcorn, incense smoke, fine clothes, and meat sacrifice. Indeed, at the end of the afternoon interview, she demanded enough funds for a chicken and a goat to sacrifice.

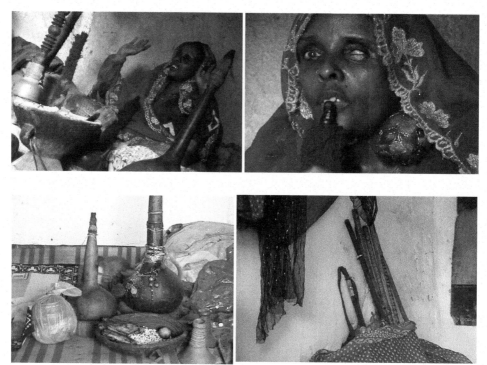

Figure 5.6 Kadija with her Jarrii Offerings and Whips

She did describe in detail her own experience with *jarrii* and how she lost her eye due to the neglect of the family *jarrii* by her father, a devout Muslim:

When I was young, the *jarrii* of my father's mother took hold of me. When my father was a young man, this *jarrii* had spoken to him and told him that it would appear again in nine years. My father, who was a devout Muslim and who had memorized the entire Qur'an during his lifetime, felt that he would be making a breach of faith if he subscribed to the worship of his mother's *jarrii*. At the age of eight, I was playing with my friends when I found that I could not see. I cried that my eyes had been taken. My family took me from doctor to doctor but still I remained blind. Finally, I was taken to Menelik Hospital in Addis and while unconscious, my *jarrii* warned: "If this doctor touches me with a knife, I will die." Those around me reported that the hospital bed began to shake violently. The doctor could not go through with the operation. Relatives warned my father that he must acknowledge the *karama* [spiritual power] of the *jarrii* that had been in our family for years and make amends. But my father grew angry, cursed the spirit, and beat me. I lost all sight in one eye but regained sight in one after several years of sacrifice. (K.A.M., April 12, 2000)

Kadija's story is typical of other tales of *jarrii* encounters. First, *jarrii* are usually inherited spirits that were important to the possessed family in the past. These spirits were provided with material goods such as libations, sacrificial meat, and perfume at annual or biannual ceremonies that took place at a memorial site in the landscape, usually at a tree or mountaintop. However, since they were neglected in subsequent generations, they make themselves heard today through the bodies of young women. The *jarrii* target young women because of their vulnerability through their excessive beauty, but the attacks themselves may also be intended to accost other members of the family – in this case, Kadija's father. Secondly, *jarrii* spirits, when unrewarded, always manifest themselves in the body first through illness. An Oromo woman from Jarso describes a typical experience with her first *jarrii* encounter:

When you first become sick with continuous headaches or heart pain, you seek out traditional medicine from a *sheik* or doctor. If you don't get better, usually someone who comes to see you will tell you to ask your family what kinds of [bad] things they've done in the past and which spirit helped them to recover. You go to the *mantiyya*. To begin with, she will give you incense medicine to see whether or not you have a *jarrii*. She will ascertain from which genealogy your *jarrii* comes. She will want to know what ceremonies your family performed in the past . . . *challee, buna qalaa, wadaajaa* . . . to ancestral spirits, and she will ask you to make sacrifices and burn incense in those same places. Then she will make preparations for a *jarrii* ceremony. Once the ceremony is performed, you can live in harmony with your spirits as long as you satisfy their desires and taboos. (M.S., March 27, 2000)

In order to identify the *jarrii,* the *mantiyya* must perform a test called '*qinii fi halluu.*' In preparation, a mixture of substances is collected by the *mantiyya* and dried and burned. This includes *qumbii, libaanata, ixaana* (incense), *quncee zuduzuu* (lemon rind), *balla ejersaa* (tree sap), *shukhaar* (spices), and *muka tinboo* (tobacco branches). During *qinii fi halluu*, the patient places her face over the stream and breathes the smoke. The patient then lies down to sleep and dream of the *jarrii* who will provide her with further instruction. If there are no such dreams, no ceremonies are performed and it is unlikely that the patient is afflicted with *jarrii*.

All *jarrii* are within the control of a *mantiyya*, who hands down her profession to her daughters. If afflicted with *jarrii*, a victim must seek out the *mantiyya* who helped her family in the past, for she will have intimate knowledge about the *jarrii*'s wants and needs. Her first action is to call to the spirit and offer incense. The person with *jarrii* will begin to shake. She may howl like a hyena while her body shakes and contorts. The afflicted is told to inhale the incense medicine, and then she is encouraged to sleep and dream. At this time, the *jarrii* is known to sing war songs about its heroic deeds and about its genealogy. Then it will let the *mantiyya* know what it wants. After this, the afflicted should become better. Then the *jarrii* ceremony is arranged. If the person doesn't perform the ceremony or doesn't do what the *jarrii* wants, she can develop leprosy, gonorrhea, or ashening of the skin. (A.A. J., April 4, 2000)

Most of the activity and all the sacrifices during the eight-day ceremony take place at night. First a hen is slaughtered, and its blood is poured over the patient. She may use leaves to wash off the blood, but no water. The next night a goat is slaughtered, and the blood is applied to her body again and cleaned with leaves and water. Then a sheep is slaughtered, and the patient is anointed with its blood. Finally, she cleans herself with leaves and water. Then all participants hold *buna qalaa* – the ritual "slaughter" of coffee beans accompanied by prayer and the drinking of coffee with butter.[51] Throughout the evenings of sacrifice, all participants drink milk. The white milk is said to cool the insides and neutralize the fierceness of the red blood.

During the ceremony, the names of powerful spirits, such as Qassaba, Halanga, Gamura, Innattii, or even Mary and Jesus, will be summoned through song and dance in order to see which spirit has taken hold of the patient. Each female member present will begin dancing in a personal manner akin to her spirit and ask for her personal objects. The room is said to become hot as each woman becomes possessed. This "hotness" is described as *merkana*, the state of feeling the effects of the chewed *khat* leaves.

In the following synopsis of the first day of the ceremony, we can begin to understand the role that Italian coins, ostrich feathers, and whip play in the ceremony:

Day 1 (Friday night): The patient and the *mantiyya* wear a white *shamma*. The *mantiyya* also wears a variety of modern gold and other metal bracelets, a necklace of yellow beads with Italian coins, and *baalli guchii* (the feather of an ostrich) in her hair. She holds a strand of *tasbii* (yellow Muslim prayer beads) in her hand. First, a cock is killed before the house door and its blood is rubbed on a big calabash. The *mantiyya* begins dancing with a *halanga* (leather whip). Later, she cuts hair from the patient's scalp, under arm, and pubic region, and clips nails from her fingers and toes. These cuttings are mixed with incense, perfume, and a little of the fermented grain with *marqaa, garbuu* (rancid or fresh butter) that will be eaten by the participants later. This bundle is tied and put inside of a calabash that will later be taken into the bush and smashed. The patient is then made to stand in the center of the room silently facing the door. In her left hand are placed eleven coins with the insignia. The patient is called by her mother's name and her *buda* enemies are cursed. A ring is placed on the fingers of the *mantiyya* and the patient to keep these enemies away. The coins are later sewn onto the patient's dress.

A *mantiyya* explains the coins:

When the Italians first came, *jarrii* went underground. Women feared the newcomers and stopped all public performances. After a few months, my grandmother, Umma Qudar, began sacrificing to her *jarrii* in public. Her *jarrii* told her she must continue with such things. People were very fearful that she would be arrested for shouting, and singing, and dancing in public. While singing, she called the names of Italian soldiers, referring to their shiny shoes decorated with metal and their coats ornamented with buttons. The Italians in Harar heard her song and brought her two boxes of their shoes. After this, everyone embraced *jarrii* practice with zeal. Since our *jarrii* liked Italians, we continue to use their coins. (K.A.M., April 14, 2000)

Indeed, the Italian Occupation (1936–1941) is today regarded as a prosperous time for Oromo people in Eastern Ethiopia during which time they were encouraged to bring back *gadaa* or *raba-dori*, their traditional governance system, reclaim land rights, and participate in mosque- and road-building projects for high wages.[52] Contrary to the Oromo experience, for urban Orthodox Christians, particularly the educated youth in Addis Ababa, the Italian Occupation is remembered as an exceptionally brutal period of international hypocrisy, eclipsed first by the death of hundreds in the Northern Highlands from mustard gas in 1936, followed by the mass assassination of 30,000 students and urban professionals in 1937. While Haile Selassie began to appeal to the League of Nations for military support in 1936, assistance by the British did not come until Italy sided with the Germans in World War II and occupied British Somaliland. The Oromo, however, saw the brief Italian period as relief from persecution by the Ethiopian state.

For this reason, *chinko*, in the form of the Maria Theresa thaler or an actual Italian coin, often adorns *jarrii* objects, particularly the ceremonial gourd pipe that is smoked during *jarrii* performances and the clothing of the participants. The shiny shoes and coat buttons also became synonymous with the Italians' ability to deflect the spiritual attacks connected to Haile Selassie. In this verse from an Oromo love song from this period, the singer praises his/her lover by comparing him/her to shiny Italian coins:

> Fine/polished/shiny
> You are a general from the city of Rome
> Fine/polished/shiny
> You are the coin made in Rome.[53]

Italian coins are used in *jarrii* both to welcome, appease, and identify the clan spirits being honored, and to bar foreign *jarrii* who are believed to be more destructive. Likewise, Italian coins are also thought to be particularly powerful in warding off *buda*. The use of foreign or colonial imagery in spirit possession parallels the connections of spirits to foreign origin as found in *Zar*, a pan-Horn of Africa phenomenon.

While the *jarrii* ceremony is described as eight days in length – a central number within Oromo genealogy and *gadaa* – it usually only lasts seven. This was explained as an influence of Islam, which favors seven and the Western calendrical system. The following is a brief synopsis of the rest of the *jarrii* ceremony:

Day 2 (Saturday): Both the patient and the *mantiyya* adorn themselves in shiny red cloth. The goats to be sacrificed are also dressed in red. When the sun sets, Innatii, the mother of all *jarrii*, and Gaamuraa are called with praise songs. These songs are sung in various languages spoken in Ethiopia. The *gayya* (gourd water pipe) and the *halanga* (whip) are tied with a cloth called '*shedare.*'

   Innatii and her mother are called through the strong aroma of pungent foods. Two hens and the red goat are killed for Innattii. Innatii requires the color red. Gaamuraa requires black.

Day 3 (Sunday): A female goat is slaughtered in the late morning and the blood is poured over the head of the patient. After sundown, a calabash is filled with honey and the spirit of Aburkas is summoned. Aburkas breaks the calabash. He requires green.

Day 4 (Monday): The spirit Addany is called. He requires *injera*, tobacco, cigarettes, and alcoholic drink. He is Christian. He requires white clothing and beads, and the sacrifice of a white sheep.

Day 5 (Tuesday): The spirit Baaba Anooroo is summoned. He requires *khat*, tobacco with ash, and *wakalimo gitoo* (stuffed intestines). He likes shiny reds and pinks. Both wear a red *foota* with gold embroidery called '*ruburubu.*'

Day 6 (Wednesday): The spirit called 'Kabir Olyaa' is summoned. He likes coffee and *khat*. He is a calm spirit also worshipped as an *awaliya*.

Day 7 (Thursday): A final sacrifice is made to Maahjaba. The red cloth with gold embroidery on the calabash and the cloth are smeared with blood. The participants also wear this cloth. The *gayya* is smoked. Everyone prays, receives blessings and then returns home.

During this ceremony, cloth of a specific color and distinct foods and smells are used to identify and please the specific spirit being honored. Innatii, venerated on Saturday, is unique as she is one of the few female-possessing spirits and she is also considered the most powerful. There are many stories about Innatii and her adventures. Of interest here is a story told by an informant in which Innatii adopts a baby with her half-sister, Atete:

   Innatii is characterized as very clever and intelligent, and she catches people's heads and causes headaches if they anger her. Her father is Muslim. Atete is associated with cattle and wealth, and her father is Amhara. Innatii was barren and Atete lost all her babies. One day, Innatii visited Atete and she brought a white baby boy. Innatii said she did not like to clean up the urine, snot, and feces, and asked her sister if she would raise the baby and give him back when he was older. Atete said that she feared the ground would eat the baby, but she agreed. Innatii made a black paste from a piece of coal and rubbed it on the baby declaring: "Let this child be black." Innatii went on to serve Sheik Hussein in the Bale region. Sheik Hussein told Innatii: "Bring the child to me but beware of crocodiles and elephants." One month later, Innatii appeared with the child and Sheik Hussein gave her a *halanga*. Sheik Hussein took the infant to a crocodile and told him to keep him until he was twelve years old. The crocodile took the baby with him into the sea and he grew up in the wild. When he reached puberty, he joined his mother and continues to travel everywhere with her. (A.A.J., April 4, 2000)

Stories and songs like this, symbolically rich in counter-narrative to proper female behavior learned during puberty, are commonly found during *jarrii* ceremonies. In this case, Innatii and Atete are barren, a condition so severe within Oromo society that it is grounds for expulsion from marriage by the husband or his family. Secondly, Innatii and Atete share a mother. In the patrilineal Oromo society where polygamy is practiced, half-siblings are always classified as sharing a father. Thirdly, the sisters reject the baby boy because they do not want to clean up after him. Among Oromo, a woman is considered irresponsible if she does not devote herself to beautifying her children or if her children appear unkempt. Lastly, the child is brought to a crocodile to be raised underwater and then later, at the age of twelve, he is given back to his mother. While the Qur'an states that *jinn* are beings created by Allah from fire, the Oromo also have a belief in *jinn*-like spirits associated with water. For this reason, women who gather water from natural springs will sometimes leave a small offering. Within proper child development, a baby boy is expected to stay in the domesticated setting under his mother's care (not underwater with crocodiles) until he nears puberty. Then he enters the domain of men, and the full-time occupation of caring for livestock and/or farming away from the domestic setting and begins to sever childhood ties with his maternal relations. In the story above, the grown boy joins Innatii and stays with her.

Such depictions of independent women who act in opposition to the ideals with which Oromo women are raised constitute a central premise in the ceremony – one that is communicated through the use of the *halanga*. The *halanga* is a man's leather whip used to control the movement of domesticated animals. During *jarrii*, those possessed by Innatii carry the *halanga* or keep it close at hand (Figure 5.6). The *halanga* invokes and identifies Innatii, and communicates the competing and inverted gender values within Oromo society through its ties to the powerful female spirit of Innatii, Sheik Hussein, and Oromo male activity.

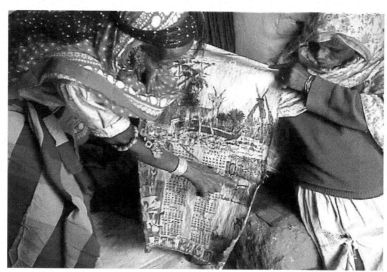

Figure 5.7 Aasha Points at an Antelope on a Kitchen Towel

Participants claim that contemporary *jarrii* practice is a modified version of the ceremony first performed during the Italian Occupation. Prior to that time, possessed adepts were said to climb onto the sacrificial antelopes or goats and sing the songs of *jarrii* while sitting on them (K.A.M., April 14, 2000). The *mantiyya* Aasha has an imported calendar towel that she keeps with her *jarrii* paraphernalia with an image of an antelope and a deer (Figure 5.7). She explained how her mother and grandmother used to ride these wild animals. Among Zar, Hauka, Shango, Shetani, Anjenu, and Bori possession practitioners, the spirit is often described as "riding" the human host. In this case, however, the women themselves are literally riding an animal before or while they themselves are ridden by the *jarrii* spirit.

When riding, some adepts say they are possessed by the spirit of Mote Qorqee, Queen of the Antelope, who, as discussed earlier, ruled through riddles, and who met an early death when she was eventually tricked and torn to pieces on the back of an antelope. The actions of Mote Qorqee, like that of the spirit Innatii, deviate from the prescribed codes of conduct within the dominant power structure of Oromo society. Through these spirits and those classified as male, women who participate in *jarrii* ceremonies and become possessed by them renegotiate how power dynamics are played out in everyday circumstances, mediate between conflicting circles, and exercise a voice that is normally ritually silent.

In this performative domain where bodies are not being protected but, instead, are made available for spirits, the need to follow prescribed conduct to repel spirits is not present. Instead, participants actively parade tension. By the manipulation of the body, prepared through costuming, props, and/or movement, a woman's identity is reconstructed to include a fusion of herself and her *jarrii* spirit. Through the use of her Janus face and body, she takes on the characteristics of the spiritual male (or anti-female) other with whom she, as an adult female, is the biological opposite. By switching codes and taking on male characteristics and objects from the male institution of *raba-dori* within this ritual frame, the adept establishes a metacommunicative language with which to articulate and bring into dialogue contradictory experiences. As Babcock (1984, 29) writes: "We seem to need a 'margin of mess,' a category of 'inverted beings' both to define and to question the orders by which we live." *Jarrii* possession can be described as role reversal, breaking prescribed societal codes, symbolic inversion, a form of play, and a way to infuse reality with actuality. From a structural–functionalist paradigm, *jarrii* as a prescribed way of behaving that deviates from one's everyday position within society, allows those with "marginal" status a means through which to vocalize their feelings during a controlled and prescribed time and space. Oromo women acknowledge that *jarrii* provides an avenue to celebrate their spirits and afford the sumptuous things not available to them during daily life. Protecting their bodies from *buda*, however, means that they must be cautious in their demeanor and defensive when choosing how to adorn themselves.

In *jarrii*, we find a range of objects and body art that is largely efficacious due to their historical or mythic affiliation. Scars incised into the skin and coins worn at the throat and forehead relate to brief historical moments of uncertainty and prosperity respectively, while ostrich feathers are distinctly imbued with the essence of *raba-dori* or *gadaa*. One of the clearest visual examples of the remnants of *gadaa* within the contemporary *jarrii* possession ceremony among the Oromo is the use of the ostrich feather, *baalli guchii*. While ostrich feathers were worn by designated men within the warrior grade between the ages of fifteen and twenty years – two among Baretuma Oromo who had demonstrated bravery – today they are worn by female possession ceremony leaders to designate their ability to placate spirits and control those with the evil eye. The transfer of a traditionally male public symbol of fearlessness to a marker of power in the private realm of spirits and women is but one way in which Oromo identity and material culture has both shifted and endured during the historical period under investigation.

Objects used in *jarrii*, including whips, feather, and knives, are also symbols of inverted womanhood, where women become associated with male behavior or possessed by spirits with male attributes. Whether serving as amulets to keep the body from the negative influences of *buda* or *jinn* or as invitations for spirits to enter the body in a controlled ceremony, these objects are used by women to take charge of negative personal forces directly affecting their lives, whether sickness or drought, whether genocide or the loss of a political voice.

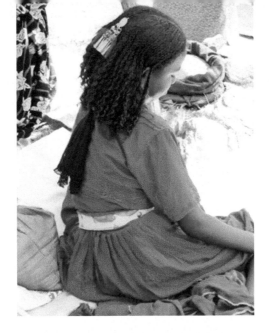

Chapter Six:

Dressing the Head in the Oromo Lifecycle

The Oromo regard the hair not only as the casing of the head, but also as a visual repository of the moral essence and life force of the individual. In this sense, the hair reflects the moral character of the individual and at different moments in life may be tightly contained, allowed to be free and unkempt or completely hidden through shaving. Each phase signals an entry into a new state of being, with its own set of moral codes that resonate metaphorically in the display of hair. This ordering of life through hair plays a key role in expressing, establishing, and maintaining identity on a personal and social level. The historical foundation for this discussion falls into the modern period, particularly the collective experiences of women since the time of the Marxist Derg government (1974–1991) and it is intended to build on the historical foundations already laid out in the previous chapters. Central concepts within the system of dress also resonate in this discussion, including notions of aesthetics and morality, gender and cosmology, tying and cutting, and revealing and containing.

Whether covered, shaved or plaited, hair is one of the first recognizable features that presents an informed observer with an accurate awareness of a woman's identity, including ethnicity, age, social standing, and marital and reproductive status. Hair in general, and its manipulations, including cutting, frizzing, and applying perfume or butter is an established practice that fluctuates very little. While I did observe that women allowed a margin of play in the length of their hair or in the length and positioning of their hairnets, these variations always fit within the referential frame of life categories.[54] Certainly, global styles are available through salon catalogues and media representations, but they are worn infrequently and only when a transnational presentation is appropriate, as when returning from a trip to Addis Ababa or from somewhere outside of Ethiopia. When asked to describe the difference between single and marital status, Oromo men and women unanimously describe the ways in which the hair is manipulated as a frame of recognition. Old women whose hair has thinned, for example, cover their sparse bundles of hair with a hairnet that sags at their shoulders like their pendulous breasts. Hair is therefore used as a public prognosis of biological maturation through its uniquely referential ability.

Hairstyle, beyond all other forms of bodily dress, traces and conveys the physical and social changes common to all women. While key components of the clothing and jewelry worn at each lifecycle stage will be mentioned, the common thread throughout this discussion of the lifecycle is the cultivation of the hair. Hairstyle and hairdressing as markers of transformation and liminality are examined through the lens of the socially marked stages that occur in a woman's life as she moves from infancy to old age: childhood and adolescence, excision, menses, marriage, and childbirth. Hair, porous and malleable, is particularly suitable as a marker for transformation due to its unique sculptural properties. Unlike the permanent practice of applying tattoos and scars, hair can be molded, teased, flattened, braided, and colored in a matter of hours, cleaned, and redressed again. If the results are still not satisfactory, hair can be cut for a new style. Since hair is constantly growing, it becomes a kind of reusable canvas that can be rearranged again and again over time. Its very nature is to change first in length throughout the prime of life and secondly in color, texture, and thickness as one nears old age.

Childhood

Oromo girls throughout Ethiopia, Kenya, and Somalia are given their first haircut as soon as they have lost their birth hair and sprouted a full head of hair. The head is then kept shaven, save for a small tuft of hair. Babies up to one year have *guttiiyyaa*, a patch of hair at the top of the forehead where the skull is soft, and the skull bones are still disconnected. *Qarree* (edge or border) is the hairstyle of breast-fed toddlers between the ages of one and three years. To create *qarree*, the center ring of hair on a girl's head is shaved, leaving a short round tuft of hair the diameter of an orange at the top of the crown called '*bantii*' ('crown of the head') and a thin outer ring of short hair along the hairline. This hairstyle is maintained by a young child's mother, who keeps the bald ring neat and tidy with a razorblade, and applies butter to her scalp to protect it from sun and dryness (Figure 6.1). This layering of a ring of hair at the crest, a ring of skin, and a final circle of hair on the crown is clearly distinct from the hairstyle of young boys.

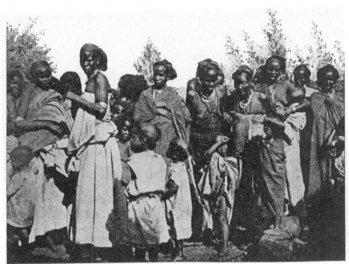

*Figure 6.1 Women with Female Children with Banti Hairstyles
(Photograph source: Rimbaud House Archives)*

Among the Wallo Oromo, after toddlerhood, boys wear *gammee*, a landing strip of hair about three inches wide from the forehead to the back of the head (Figure 6.2). *Gammee* refers to a *gadaa* age grade when boys wear their hair short on the sides with a patch of hair at the crest. As they enter the Raab Grade, a small tonsure is left on the crown, the rest of the hair grows long, and they may marry. As the hair grows long and erect in Mohawk style, it is braided or twisted into dreadlock and called '*guduru*.' The shaved borders are still referred to as '*qarree*' until seven to ten years of age. Then the *gomfee* (wild teenage hair) starts when a young man begins to comb and butter his full coiffure. At this time, the boy is said to be 'out of *gammee*,' and he takes on new responsibilities and begins to consider marriage.

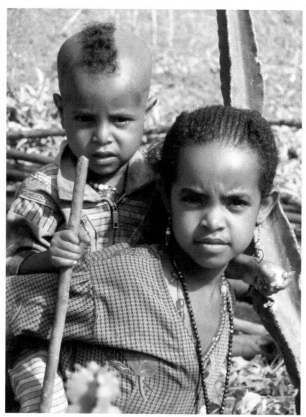

Figure 6.2 Wallo Boy with Gammee Hairstyle

Among the Afran Qallo, boys wear their head shaved entirely, except for a small round patch of hair at the top or front of the crown about the size of a tangerine. This hairstyle is called '*tuttoo*,' the name given to a clump of tall grasses that the hairstyle resembles and also a derivative of *tutuma*, the name for the comb of a cock. The boys' hairstyle is considered the visual ideal in the Oromo masculine idiom for several reasons. First, informants state that the projection of hair just above the forehead is considered a precursor to the metal, phallic headpiece worn by adult men in the past and known as '*kallicha*' (Figure 6.3) (A.K., March 27, 2000; M.S., March 27, 2000). In *gadaa* or *raba-dori*, the Oromo Kallu or moiety head was also a divine mediator and his position was visually communicated by the *kalaacha* or *kallicha* (Baxter and Almagor 1987, 167). While most Barentuma leaders have not worn the *kallicha* regularly in over one hundred years, the practice can still be observed among the Arsi and southern Boraana Oromo. The *kallicha* may be connected to the ancient practice of the wearing of the genitals of a fallen enemy on the forehead by the killer or placing them around the neck of the killer's spouse or on the door of his home. This practice of castration of male enemies was reported by Paulitschke (1893, 92) to have harnessed the secretive, procreative ability of the deceased as among the Rendille and Samburu pastoralists in Kenya (Spencer 1973,

52, 97). During *gadaa*, Oromo men, ready to take on the role of elders, shaved their erect warrior hairstyle and substituted the phallic *kallicha*. While the *tuttoo* hairstyle for young boys and adolescents is shared by other ethnic groups, the visual connections to the *kallicha* as well as to the erect tufts that warriors wore in the past, makes this hairstyle unique from that of other Ethiopian boys.

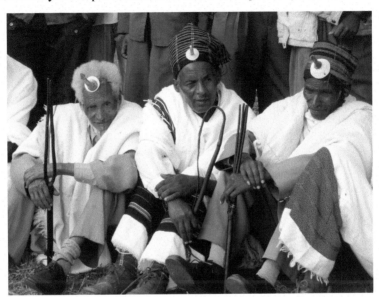

Figure 6.3 Arsi Men wearing Kallicha

Informants claim that this erect style was adopted by the Oromo only within the last fifty years in an attempt to visually recreate the idealized male hair preparation and dressing during the time of *raba-dori*, stating that drawing on memories and stories of warriorhood instills a sense of Oromummaa in a young boy (M.R.A., February 20, 2000; I.A., May 6, 2010). The linguistic connection to tall grasses also relays his community's hopes that he will bring about abundant harvest as a farmer and/or raise large herds through his ability to supply ample nourishment to his animals. More generally, and true among the Amhara as well, the linguistic and visual associations with the cock's comb is also connected to aspirations of virility.

While a small boy may be affectionately called a 'little rooster' with a fine crest sprouting on his head – a crest that will someday stand erect and proud – the hairstyle of a girl is associated with her future livelihood as mother and household overseer. The circles of hair and bare scalp compare to the layout of a homestead, where a wattle-and-thatch hut is protected by a thorn fence or stone wall. More specifically, the round tuft at the center of the head may also be referred to as 'her mother's navel or nipple', suggesting, on the one hand, her dependency on her mother for nurture while in the womb and after birth and, on the other hand, her own future procreative capacity (R.M.O., March 6, 2000). For a baby girl, hair is already infused with her ties to her maternal group and her reproductive capacities.

The shift away from the distinctive markings of rings of hair next to a ring of exposed scalp during later childhood signals a girl's departure from the more liminal period of infancy when an infant is particularly vulnerable to illness, disease, and spiritual harm associated with *buda*. Sieber (2000, 16) attributes the tuft of hair left at the front of the crown among small children throughout Africa to serving a protective function against harmful spirits. This is true, to some extent, in the Horn of Africa. If someone afflicted with the evil eye becomes jealous of the beauty of a newborn, for example, the baby can die. Owing to one of the highest infant mortality rates in the world, Oromo babies have only a seventy percent chance of survival. This rate decreases drastically after the fourth or fifth year, when hair is usually allowed to grow long. Head hair, particularly when it is long and greasy with butter, may attract the unwanted attention of spirit-inflicted sickness or biting insects, so mothers maintain the short cut until around the age of five years, when "they are completely mobile and can scratch their own heads" (I.M., November 10, 2001). Once the hair fills in, mothers begin placing shiny metal or beaded ornaments in their children's hair to protect it from *buda* by deterring attention away from the hair itself. This is also done to beautify the hair until it is long enough to be properly braided. These first hair ornaments play the same role as metal and beaded necklaces, and facial scars for a young girl – to invite attention through the enhancement of form and to protect through minor alterations or disfigurements in order to conceal her natural beauty. The belief that "natural beauty," a body attribute that has not been socially altered, is particularly vulnerable to damaging spirits or jealous humans is a central theme within the Oromo aesthetic system. In the case of head hair, the "natural" hair at childhood is protected either through the removal or application of cosmetics. Since the hair is said to encapsulate the vitality of the child and infant death is a major concern, shielding the scalp and hair from magical attack is a central anxiety for new mothers. A variety of herbs, amulets, and decorations are often added to the head to protect it.

As baby girls reach the age of five or six years, the bald areas of their *banti* are no longer maintained and their hair can grow in naturally. In this state, when the hair is no longer shaved, girls are affectionately referred to as 'little women.' This growing-out stage is allowed to continue without further cutting of the hair for three to four years. Only when the hair has reached several inches in length is it neatly combed from the forehead and a shiny chain or a bright piece of string is placed on the head to keep the hair from the eyes of the wearer. The Karayyu and other pastoralists like the Arsi use leather bands for this purpose. A proverb explains that once the bareheaded *banti* style has grown out, the parents of the girl begin taking inquiries and gifts from the families of potential husbands for their daughter. Similarly, in the late 1880s, Paulitschke (1893, 107) mentions that in Harar, Oromo girls wear a bald spot to indicate that they are not yet ready to have offspring. In this sense, the end of the shaved style and the subsequent hair growth marks a girl's preparation for engagement and married life. Similarly, it is said that when an Oromo man loses all his hair at an advanced age, he moves from procreative potential to impotence. Baldness in both cases indicates a chaste self.

Among Oromo today, when the bald area of the *banti* style has grown in and the hair surrounding this circular spot reaches a few inches in length, the hair is twisted or braided (Figure 6.4). A discussion of hair and adolescence anywhere in Ethiopia (or Africa, for that matter) would be incomplete without mentioning the braid. Girls and young women throughout the country wear braids in a variety of styles and thicknesses. If the braids are executed very thinly, they are called '*nannoo*.' *Nannoo* refers to a young woman's hairstyle throughout the Barentuma Oromo homeland. The hair is divided along a middle part and braids or plaits are created by vertically braiding three divisions of hair usually while gathering bits of hair along the way in order to keep the braids close to the scalp. This braided hairstyle called '*nannoo*' in Afan Oromo (*shurrubba* among Amharic speakers, *guruz* in the Semitic Argobba language, *Harari gruss* in the Harari language). It is found in all regions of Ethiopia without exception.

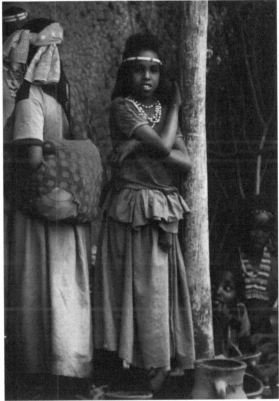

Figure 6.4 Girl in Baabile with Tuft of Hair at Crown of Head

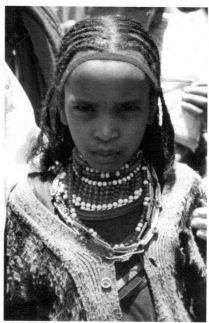

Figure 6.5 Girl in Jarso with Nanno Hairstyle and Red Yarn at Hairline

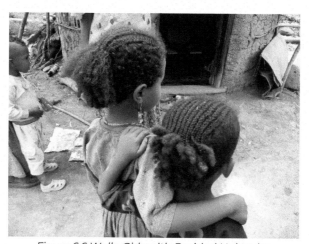

Figure 6.6 Wallo Girls with Braided Hairstyles

Once all the hair along the vertical path has been incorporated into the braid, the remaining portion is allowed to hang loosely to the ears, framing the face (Figure 6.5). This bottom portion of the braid may be left loose, braided further or separated into two pieces and twisted together. Among the Karrayyu and Ittu, the hair along the part is twisted, in a style known as '*daabee*' with a shorter step in the back (*madho*). While Afran Qallo girls continue to let their hair grow during adolescence, they usually keep the hair on the crown short and unbraided so that this clump of hair stands high on the crown (Figure 6.4). This hairstyle, *nannoo bantii,* is in marked contrast to the style of young girls in Wallo, who let the top knot grow while keeping the sides short (Figure 6.6).

The combination of braids and *banti* in *nannoo bantii* indicates a girl's physical and social maturation. She has already learned and is often responsible for primary household duties, including cleaning, collecting water, shopping, preparing the coals for cooking, and making tea and coffee for her family and their guests. However, she has not experienced the two significant events necessary for womanhood: (1) the onset of menses and (2) her excision ceremony. Her childhood *banti* coupled with her adolescent braids reminds her and others that this is soon to come.

The act of aestheticizing the hair is taught to girls by respected female elders. An Oromo girl typically receives the *nannoo bantii* when she is between the ages of eight and ten years from an Ogeetii, a woman well versed in medicinal and cultural practices, including the preparation of traditional medicines and midwifery. A young woman from Baabile recounts her first braided hairstyle:

> My mother took me to the Ogeetii and she placed my head in her lap. The Ogeetii divided my hair equally down the middle and began to make small, tight braids with three strands of hair: first on the right side of my head and then on the left. This process is referred to as '*dhawachu.*' I tried to remember each step in my mind. When she neared the bottom, she twisted the hair together and applied fresh butter from the root of a bamboo shoot. My mother paid her, and she took me out to dance *shuguyyee* and show off my new hairstyle. (M.M., March 25, 2000)

If the braids are thick and less numerous than *nannoo,* they are often referred to as '*shurrubba Oromo.*' *Shurrubba* is an Amharic term that refers specifically to the braided hairstyle in which the remaining hair at the bottom of the thick braid is further divided. These divisions are also braided, and they create branch-like projections that fan out from the face. This style is particularly suitable for dancing. During dances in which young women jerk their torsos to and fro, and wave their heads back and forth, the braided hairstyle is activated. This pendulum of head and hair is meant to draw attention to the beauty of the dancer's neck and to show off her grace and agility. The more her head and shoulders quiver in the performance, the more spectacularly her braids will fly and the more praise she will receive from the audience.

The creation of *nannoo banti* and *Oromo shurrubba* hairstyles is described by women as similar to the process of basket making. While the plaiting on Oromo baskets is in technique quite different than braiding, both are loosely categorized as weaving strands of material over and under to create distinct patterns. This style of wear began in the early nineteenth century when most settled Oromo communities were engaging full time in agriculture and women began plaiting baskets. Hence, even among agricultural communities there is a clear association of men's hair with cattle herding and the wild, and women's hair with the domestic realm and agriculture. There is a visual sense of the orderly containment of hair in contrast with the *Gomfee* hairstyle of men, which is natural and buttered (Figure 6.7).

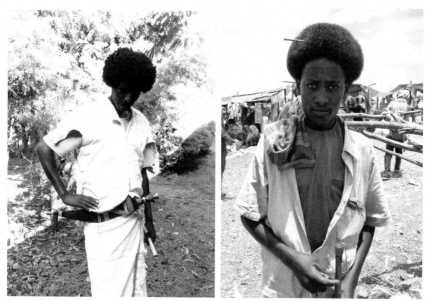

Figure 6.7 Young Wallo Men with Gomfee Hairstyle

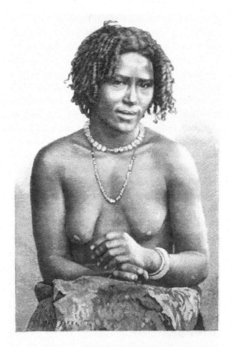

JEUNE FILLE GALLA
D'après une photographie de M. P. Soleillet et L. Chefneux.

Figure 6.8 Oromo Pastoralist wearing Martuu Hairstyle
(Source: Reclus 307)

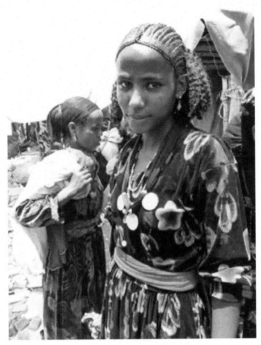

Figure 6.9 Wallo Woman's Hairstyle

It should be mentioned that prior to the Derg period, Oromo women who lived in traditionally pastoralist communities in Baabile and Fedis wore a hairstyle called '*martuu*' or '*mataa*,' popular among all Oromo groups at the turn of the century (Figure 6.8). To create *martuu*, the hair is first divided down the middle and then separated into two bundles. These divisions are segmented into two strands of hair that are rubbed between the hands to twist the strands around each other. The twists hang down the sides of the head and are secured with red clay and a thin leather band to keep the hair out of the eyes. When dancing, this band is removed so that the hair also splays outward, with length and fullness indicating the age of the dancer.

In Wallo, unmarried women's hairstyles are strongly influenced by the styles worn by Tigrayan women, including French-braided sections of hair from the crown to just beyond the top of the head. The uniqueness of Wallo Oromo hairdressing is the braided strand anchored across the forehead, created by bringing the thickest braided hair along the central part forward and then across the forehead (Figure 6.9). This braid acts as a forehead binder in the same way that asparagus fiber and leather keep the hair in place in other Barentuma areas. In Tigre, women add a silver ornament to this space and among the Afar, a button.

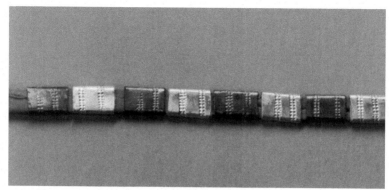

Figure 6.10 Addoo Forehead Band made with Copper and Tin

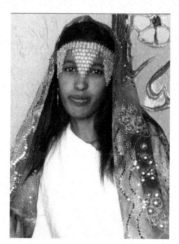

Figure 6.11 Qarmaa Loti

Historically, decoration of the head with supplemental ornaments differed between agriculturalists and pastoralists just as hairstyles did. Among agriculturalists, the forehead was tied with *addoo* or *aadata* made from grain fibers, ideally barley, and worn by young women. The grain stalk was cut into small rectangular pieces that were strung onto fiber or the *meedicha* leather strap. A modern version of this forehead band where the *addoo* is fashioned from copper and tin beads strung on a leather cord is housed in the collection of the Institute of Ethiopian Studies Museum in Addis Ababa (Figure 6.10). Among pastoralists, in contrast, a leather forehead band was worn called '*dhihee*' (or '*dhi'ee*'). *Dhihee* was made from cow or sheep skin cut into a thick strip and dyed red with a plant extract. While all Oromo girls and women wore the dress of white sheeting, *saddetta*, the grain *addoo* and the leather *dhihee* communicated the wearer's livelihood, locality, and the goods that she might be carrying in her pastoral community.

In the last fifty years when they could afford it, Oromo women in both farming and herding villages began replacing their fiber and leather headbands with metal forehead bands known collectively as '*qarmaa*.' The most common *qarmaa*, called '*qarmaa loti*' (chain headband) consists of a silver, metal mesh strand (Figure 6.11).

The more elaborate *qarmaa loti,* reserved for special occasions among the Afran Qallo, is fashioned into five triangles. These metal forehead pieces are created by Harari smiths in Harar, and sold in the gold and silver shops in the old horse market, Faras Magala. The wealthier Harari, who also make and wear *qarmaa loti* (called '*siyassa*' by the Harari), reproduce seven triangles instead of five and use gold instead of silver or other alloys. When placed side by side, an Oromo woman's *qarmaa loti* looks different from the mesh piece worn by the Harari woman (Figure 6.12). Both women wear *qarmaa* but the one is made of interlocking pieces of nickel and tin, while the one is made of gold alloy and is more intricate.

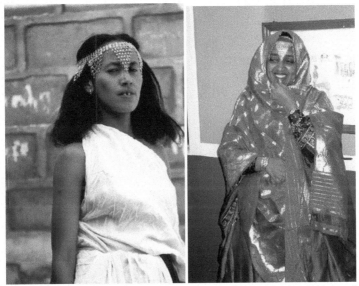

Figure 6.12 (Left) An Oromo Woman's Qarmaa Loti (Right) A Harari Woman's Siyassa

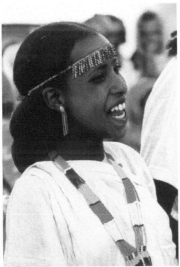

Figure 6.13 An Afran Qallo Woman wearing Qarmaa Loti fashioned from Manufactured Metal Chain

In the 1970s, pre-made spools of low-grade metal chain began arriving in the marketplace and local Oromo recreated *qarmaa loti* with this new readymade material (Figure 6.13). This industrial material was cheap, readily available and, most importantly, Oromo women no longer had to enter Harari jewelry shops where they were often made to feel like second-class citizens. In the last fifteen years, this metal headpiece has been transformed again through a network of colorful seed beads that are either worn with the spool *qarmaa loti* or have replaced it entirely. This modern beaded band is called '*challee qarmaa*' (beaded headpiece). *Challee qarmaa* refers to both open interlaced strands of multicolored seed beads and horizontal strands of white seed beads connected with plastic, colored buttons. The latter is worn mostly in Fedis and referred to as '*bishanni*', from *bishan*, meaning 'water,' due to the predominately white beads that are characterized as clear, glistening and watery in color. *Bishanni* are worn on market days and on special occasions, when young girls seek to be attractive and accentuate their shiny black hair. They are also an indication of a young girl's popularity, as the beads used in the making of *bishanni* are often given by potential suitors to the girls they admire.

Challee qarmaa and *bishanni qarmaa* worn with the seed bead necklaces that resemble these beaded headbands create a complete set of upper body jewelry (Figure 6.14). While earrings made of seed bead loops and other necklaces may be added, and exposed arms may be decorated with tin bracelets, they serve as secondary items to the crucial placement of beaded forehead and necklace bands. Each woman takes great pride in the purchase, production, and wear of these materials. Women I spoke with explained that it took several hours to complete their *challee* (beadwork). Since the beadwork itself is not difficult, women are able to produce their *challee* themselves and while they may work in groups when they have a free moment in the day, they try to differentiate their own *challee* from others through individual choices in patterning and color. It is considered a shameful offense to copy the designs of others or to sell or trade one's necklace. When a woman dies, her daughters will cut and unravel her necklaces and headbands, and distribute the beads for future jewelry rather than wear the *challee* or save it as a memento. Beaded bands, then, have a lifecycle dependent on the life span of their owner. When I asked why *challee* could not be exchanged (hoping to buy one myself) women laughed and I was told: "When the body dies it goes back to the earth. When the beads die, they go back to other bead work" (J.A., February 3, 2000).

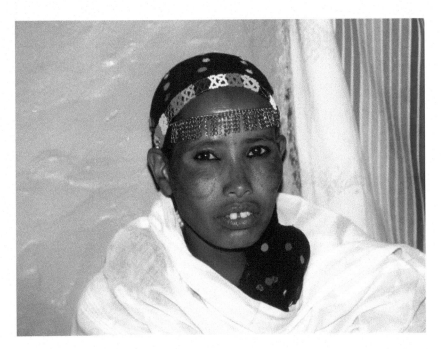

Figure 6.14 An Afran Qallo Woman wearing Gufta Bombei, Qarmaa Loti, and Challee Qarmaa

Challee worn on the forehead and at the neck functions as a statement about a woman's financial position, her capacity as a skilled artisan and weaver, and her desire to accentuate and draw attention to her torso and head. By extension, unmarried women further advertise their skills and mark their interest in future mates through the necklaces they bead for young men (Figure 6.15). Lastly, the distinctive diamond-shaped patterns and primary colors of beaded headbands and necklaces also signal a more personal transformation of the wearer herself. While girls may wear a single beaded strand, young women begin wearing complete beaded sets after their excision ceremonies. And at the onset of menses, which usually follows this earlier rite, young women receive strands of beads from their relatives and are encouraged to bead while they sit in seclusion.

Young girls are encouraged to keep their hair sweet smelling, adding perfumed plants and oils. Among the Wallo in Bati, *arrittii*, an aromatic plant, is inserted into the hair and worn in a metal ring pinned to a girl's chest. When girls and boys engage in a call and response of riddles, a girl who fails to respond inserts her *arrittii* into a chosen boy's hair to signal her affection. The girl's locks are also buttered with powdered leaves (*addis*) leaving the hair green and shiny.

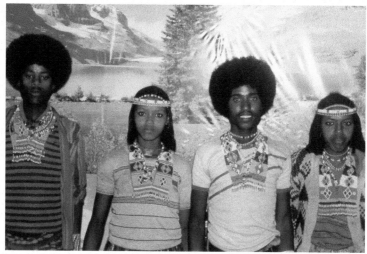

Figure 6.15 Young Oromo Men and Women wearing Beaded Ambarka and Sex-Specific Hairstyles. Source: Harar Photo Studio

Puberty and Menstruation

Hairstyles and hairdressing are visual cues that communicate a girl's developing body during the years prior to and during puberty. They also signal the more hidden, cultural changes that accompany sexual maturation: genital cutting. While this topic is sensitive, especially for readers unaccustomed to the practice, excision is viewed as part of the continuum of body art practice that make a girl a woman. Oromo women I spoke with felt it was a necessary part of their coming-of-age experience and not a topic to shy away from. It is included in this chapter as it relates to dressing the head during puberty.

To signify a young woman's readiness for womanhood and marriage, some Oromo girls undergo one of two forms of genital cutting or a combination of the two – either *absuma arabi* (excision of the prepuce of the clitoris and, in most cases, the partial sewing of the inner labia) or *absuma hodha* (the full removal of the clitoris, parts of the labia majora and the labia minora, and the sewing together of the remnants of the labia minora. The cutting is further a symbol of containment that both promotes the sexual maturity of the young woman while harnessing her sexuality. During the historic practice of *absuma hodha* or Pharaonic circumcision (which today has been outlawed by Shari'a law and is only practiced regularly among Somali women or Oromo women who are engaged to Somali men), the patient has her whole body ritually cleansed, her head shaved, and her nails cut to mark her transformation. This "baldness" signifies her healing period and her inability to marry, for a woman must have hair to become a wife.[55] The Oromo state that they did not practice female circumcision prior to the 1800s and Paulitschke (1893, 174–175) in the 1880s reports that *absuma arabi* was only practiced by devote Muslims. The Afran Qallo say that *absuma hodha* was introduced by Muslim proselytizers and later enforced in the east by the Egyptian Government at the end of the nineteenth century.[56]

During the modern procedure of *absuma arabi,* also referred to as '*dhagna qabaa*' in the north (literally 'to catch the body'), the shaving of hair is no longer practiced, but hair still plays a central, symbolic role in a young woman's healing process. At the onset of the contemporary ceremony, a girl's female relatives remove her braids. This unraveling of braids and the subsequent bushy appearance of the hair signals a state in which the body is vulnerable and thereby "uncontained." This unruly hair is worn only when a woman's body has undergone major trauma, including childbirth and the surgery of *absuma arabi.*

For *absuma arabi* the Ogeetii is called to bring *haaduu shanta* (a very sharp thing). The patient sits against an upside-down *mooyyee* (a large wooden bowl used for grinding). Two women hold her arms at her sides or they are tied to the *mooyyee.* Her legs are also bound – the left leg is tied to or held by the woman on her left and her right leg by the woman on her right. When her limbs are secured, the Ogeetii severs the hood of the clitoris with a knife and makes two small incisions above and below this area. If necessary, she rubs a mixture of ground herbs on the wound to control the bleeding. Thorns tied with thread are inserted through these cuts. During the healing process, the skin is meant to close over the area of the truncated clitoris and, after three days, the threaded thorns are eventually pulled free. While I refer to the procedure of *absuma arabi* as an excision, the focus of the operation is not merely on removing the clitoris. Instead, the cutting is regarded as a necessary step in order to create a smooth covering over the upper opening of the vagina. Paulitschke describes a very similar process among the neighboring Somali and Afar in the 1880s whereby the clitoris and labia minor are cut away, the remaining skin is sewn together with horsetail thread, and the application of incense smoke and a salve made of the jojoba plant are administered in the healing process.

When she removes the thorns, the Ogeetii adds a mixture of tree resin and powdered kohl to the wound. This mixture is intended to aid in the healing process and blacken the skin. The patient is not allowed to drink milk, and she eats only a mixture of wheat and barley called '*qinxa*' with butter and dried meats. The purpose of the tattooing of the upper outer labia after the operation could not be easily explained by the women I spoke with. Some women dismissed it as merely medicinal, while others mentioned that it beautified the area by turning a "red" area "black." A similar explanation is given throughout Ethiopia for the tattooing of the upper gums among women from a variety of ethnic groups. The black color hides the pink gums and brings out the whiteness of the teeth. Pink gums are thought to be unattractive, and informants went so far as to call the color shameful. The blackening of the vaginal skin during *absuma arabi* may also be intended to keep harmful spirits who are captivated by bloodshed and bodily openings at bay, as Boddy (1989) observed among Muslim women in northern Sudan.[57]

After the operation, a *sabbata* (belt) is used to bind the initiate's legs during the healing period, keeping her from walking and allowing her wound to heal. During sleep, her big toes are also tied together with a strip of cloth. The type of *sabbata* used to bind the legs is called '*manqux*.' As Oromo women do not wear constricting or concealing pants, they say that the tight feeling of the cloth is something constantly in their minds during this liminal healing period. Once they marry, the *sabbata* will bind their waists and be kept hidden underneath the folds of their dress, hiding and enclosing the home of a future fetus. While healing, girls are advised to think about their genealogy or, more specifically, "the ties that bind them to their family," as they experience the taut sensation at their thighs and the pain of the wound.

Along with their honeymoons and the days prior to childbirth, the weeks after excision are a period of inactivity unknown during normal life when women are usually very preoccupied with their daily domestic and commercial tasks. Women tell me that their immobility coupled with the rhythmic, smarting sensations at their legs and vagina create an altered or hypnotic state of being that allows them to investigate new ideas, often spiritual in nature, without interruption. In some cases, women reported that it was during their seclusion that they first encountered their *jarrii* spirits. As is the case among initiates in most rites of passage, this extraordinary event is often offered to young women as a time of reflection on spiritual connections, generative potential, and their future role as wives.

Newly circumcised girls are joined by female relatives who visit them in their homes with gifts of cloth and beads, sing to them, tell them stories about their clan histories and family spirits, and brush and oil their hair. While visitors do not directly see the healing process of the wound, they may examine the length and texture of the hair of the circumcised girl as a sign of her progress. Since it has not been cut some weeks prior to her surgery or during her recovery, her hair will have grown. In this way, long hair on the crown that has fully covered the exposed scalp she wore as a young girl comes to stand for the tattooed skin that has closed around the clitoral area. In both cases, an area on the body associated with childhood has been covered or hidden. This is a necessary physical procedure in order to visually create the notion of Oromo womanhood.

When girls were excised prior to the onset of menstruation, menses usually follows within a few years. At this time, her hair should have grown long and full, and she will be ready to marry. During marriage, the *sabbata* that was once wound tightly across her thighs during her seclusion is now placed by female relations around her waist.[58] Today, in the most heavily Islamized regions, the operation takes place when an Oromo girl is much younger – up to one week after birth for both girl and boy babies. In Wallo, the Amharic term '*girrizat*' is used for the operation, which includes the cutting away of the clitoris and labia minora. It is expected to heal without sewing. The use of the Amharic term suggests this practice may have come from the outside and adopted within the last three generations.

The transfer of the cloth from the legs to the waist is significant. During circumcision, the *sabbata* is integrally connected to the closing of the vagina by the Ogeetii. When placed at the waist, the sash alludes to the opening of the vagina both as an entrance for the husband's penis and as an outlet for future babies and then closed. The sash carries with it the fundamental notion of the opening and closing of the sex, and the pain experienced in each of those endeavors. Wrapped at the waist in the manner of the Great Mothers, the *sabbata* also bears the symbolic responsibility of reproducing the descendants of Barentu and the four sons of Qallo. For those familiar with the *sabbata's* associations, a waist bound with cloth is, above all, an indication of a fertile womb.

If we turn again to the song from Fedis, the contrast between the male singer's head and that of the girl he describes is evident:

> The sack of coffee is taken to one's house,
> The silver that is loved is taken overseas.
> You tied beads together for your forehead,
> One is interlocked with another.
> And you tied your stomach with cloth,
> But my head and stomach are shaking for you.[59]

This passage discusses the binding and, hence, controlling of a woman's beauty at the waist and forehead while the male protagonist's own forehead and stomach shake seemingly out of control. This song also contrasts metaphorically the visual differences in hairstyle and behavior among men and women. Young men's hair is ideally full and visually unruly during young adulthood relating back to a pastoral livelihood in which young men were living outside of the village in closely knit fraternities with others of their age group and engaging full-time in hunting, cattle herding, cattle raiding, and, as one Oromo elder put it, "applying butter to their wild hair" (I.A., February 20, 2000). Their hairstyle between the ages of fifteen and twenty-two years is called '*dhumfura*' – a high afro with the bottom shaved straight across and maintained with the prodding of a circular wooden stick. To keep its shape, fat, butter and wax were used on the hair, and a headrest kept the hairstyle intact when men were resting or sleeping. Despite the great effort that was generated to create and preserve these styles, their frizziness was intended to suggest ferocity and the untamed. Warriors throughout Ethiopia have used their hair as a marker of their power and prestige. During periods of war in the past, as men gathered in forested areas for military training, their hair could not be properly cared for. This matted and dreaded style became an indicator of a man's training in the wilderness and his ability to withstand the comforts of family life. His hair also alluded to the temporarily dangerous period of war, likely marked by bloodshed and tragedy. Coming across this young man might intimidate his enemy and alert his compatriots that they should seek safety. Young girl's hair, in contrast, is tightly contained close to the scalp through their braided hairstyles and the interlocking beaded bands that keep their hair flat. This differing aesthetic of the hair of young men and young women is clearly illustrated in Figure 6.15, where four young people wearing beaded necklaces stand side by side; the girls with flat braided hair held in place with *bishanni qarmaa* and the boys with high, teased afros that make them appear much taller than they really are.

Men also shake and flaunt their hair while dancing, as the term 'head shaking' in the song alludes. A successful dancer is able to move his shoulders in small pulsations that seem to ripple down his torso while his legs propel his body gracefully up and down. This movement is broken with interludes of jumping when the head is flicked to and fro to draw particular attention to the wild beauty of the hair. While women also engage in the fanning of their braids during dancing in adolescence, once their braids are removed at excision and they later marry, they no longer wear these braids or dance with the same vigor.

The line about the tying of beads together on the forehead in the song (while the silver that once decorated the forehead is taken overseas) also illustrates the importance of adornment during this life stage. Young single women and those married only a few years are the most elaborately decorated, particularly on their hair, ear, neck, and upper torso. When asked why young women wear such a display of jewelry, Afran Qallo women explained time and again: "To be a woman demands beads." Womanhood as a cultural category has a natural and cultural association with blood – the blood loss connected to excision through the intervention of human actors, on the one hand, and monthly menstruation dependent on the lunar cycle, on the other. Since blood is considered particularly attractive to harmful spirits, the association of womanhood with blood makes women more susceptible to supernatural aggression than men and they are especially vulnerable during their monthly cycle. In this sense, the strands of beads on the hair, ears, and neck that surround, frame, and call attention to the face are also meant to detract from the immediacy of the face and harness the harmful evil eye.

Absuma arabi is ideally performed a couple of years prior to the beginning of menses – between the ages of eight and ten years. Unlike boys' circumcision to which the community is alerted and invited for gift-giving and feasting, the girl's excision is a more private affair that is only attended by immediate matrilineal female relatives. The onset of menses is similarly observed. Women usually remember the first day of menstruation as a pivotal moment when their mothers and sympathetic older female relatives joined together and cared for them in their homes. Some women told me that their mothers tied red cotton thread to their foreheads, gave them milk to drink, and told them the story about the origins of menstrual blood (S.Y., February 14, 2000; I.M., May 29, 2010).

One myth common among the Barentuma Oromo states that when the world began, it was men who menstruated, and women who administered all ritual and political affairs. When men menstruated, they bled from their foreheads on a lunar cycle. One day, a kindly sister wiped the flow of blood from her brother's forehead. Through this act, she took the blood from him and she began to bleed from her own body. From that day onward, women started menstruating. In her classic work on women and myth, Bamberger (1974, 276) states that stories of a distant and tumultuous past when women were in control is a common model for explaining why it is that men should hold positions of power today. The Oromo myth fits within this paradigm. The story as it was told to me, however, also stresses the procreative ability that men once held but was later taken from them by women.

To remember this historical moment, the story goes, women in future generations tied red yarn to their foreheads when they bled, while men adopted the *kallicha*, their phallic head ornament (Figure 6.3). The *kallicha* was intended to disguise the place from which they bled (M.M., March 5, 2000). This area at the center of the forehead is still considered an extremely vulnerable place for men. Whether men associate the *kallicha* with this myth is not something I could ascertain, since it has not been worn regularly in several generations. Among the southern Boraana Oromo who practice *gadaa* in an abbreviated form and where the *kallicha* is still worn, some insights can be gleaned about its associations with women. When a Boraana man reaches the grade of *gadaamoojii* (full retirement), he wears *kallicha* and is referred to by the female pronoun (Kassam and Megersa 1989, 29). While the association of the forehead with menstrual blood is also not evident from scholarly accounts of the Borana, the practice of wearing the *kallicha* during retirement is connected to Oromo femininity, and associated with peaceful relations and the domestic realm. This is not unlike the wearing of a woman's *gufta* and *saddetta* (hairnet and dress) by Oromo male council leaders traveling to see Abba Muuda. They are worn then to communicate their humility and promote harmonious relations, highlighting women's perceived role as natural peacemakers.

Whether or not the Borana example is relevant to the Barentuma today, what is significant to this discussion is the mention made of the covering of the area that bled in the menstruation myth. In a similar manner, the sealing up and darkening of the female sex during excision may also be intended to hide or protect a vulnerable area associated both with blood and procreation. Among pastoralist Somali, for example, Talle (1993, 86) reports that there is a clear association between the frequent viewing of the genitals and blindness. If one considers Oromo excision from this viewpoint, it is not the genitals that are being protected, but, rather, it is the human gaze that is being shielded from a powerful and dangerous area associated with the flow of blood. In this reading, the closed, tattooed skin is a way to protect the eye from the vagina. I hesitate to bestow too much weight on this explanation of excision, however, since it was never orally communicated in this way.

Just as the story of Mote Qorqee explains why women do not hold political office, the story of the red yarn explains why women bleed – two states that were mythically reversed among men and women in the mythic past. Today, these red threads are still worn but they are placed on the forehead to accentuate the hair (Figure 6.5). Paulitschke (1888a) reports that neighboring Afar warriors tied red silk threads around their foreheads when they had killed someone, in this case to symbolize the spilling of blood. Among the Oromo, there is no longer a clear correspondence between the yarn forehead band and bloodshed or the state of menses. Women do adorn their hair, however, with certain herbs when they have their periods. These herbs, unlike the red yarn, are intended to be hidden. Odiferous plants such as myrrh, thyme, and garlic cloves may be inserted into the hairnet or tucked into the back of the hair to give off a pungent smell that is designed to deflect or placate harmful spiritual forces such as *jinn* and *jarrii* who are particularly drawn to women during menses. Further, these herbs also work as a kind of non-verbal, non-visual communication to a husband who may come to her for sex. Since there is a strong belief that diseases such as gonorrhea and human immunodeficiency virus (HIV) are contracted through sex practiced during menses, the pungent odor coming from the hairnet or *gufta* allows men to avoid sexual encounters that they perceive as risky. From a woman's perspective, this perfume may allow temporary repose from her husband's sexual advances.

The Married Woman's *Gufta*

As we learned in the antics of the ruthless fabled leader Mote Qorqee in Chapter Four, that which makes a woman powerful are her breast and her hairnet (the loss of both immobilizes Mote Qorqee). The most crucial element of a married woman's costume has been, by tradition, her *gufta*. A *gufta* is an imported, black, net hair covering used by most Barentuma Oromo women. To wear *gufta*, the unbraided hair is parted down the middle. This is referred to as' *banti baqassa*' and the husband may affectionately refer to his new bride as '*bantitiqo*' ('my *banti*') as her hair is parted for him when he becomes her husband. It is then either braided or, in the case of the Afran Qallo, pulled back to form two balls, tied at the nape of the neck, and covered with netting (Figure 6.16). This hairstyle in the Eastern Highlands of Ethiopia is known as '*hamasha*.' Underneath the *gufta*, a thin fiber headband called '*miggaaja*' is tied to keep the hair in place. On top of the *gufta* other headbands called '*naasi*' among the Afran Qallo or '*shaashii*' among the Wallo are laid down to secure the *gufta* (Figure 6.17). Newly married Arsi women place a plethora of ornaments over their *gufta*, to the point where it is difficult to see (Figure 4.3). By menopause, the forehead ornaments have disappeared and are replaced with a white cloth band tied over this black hairnet.

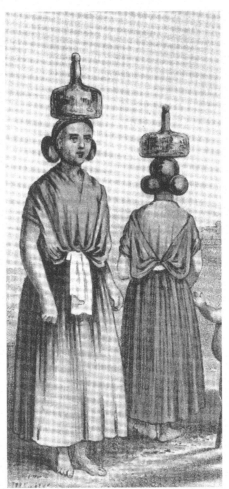

Figure 6.16 Drawing of Harari Women wearing Gufta (Source: Burton 1987, 16 vol.II)

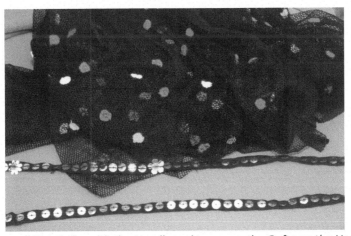

Figure 6.17 A Gufta with the Nassii used to secure the Gufta on the Head

Oromo women in villages such as Fedis and Jarso claim that *gufta* has only been worn there for two generations. Other Oromo groups say that it was adopted with the introduction of Islam to the northeastern region.[60] Since we know from Burton's illustrations that urban women were wearing *gufta* as early as the 1850s, it is likely that *gufta* wearing originated in Harar and was adopted outward to more distant areas. One particular kind of *gufta*, *gufta bombei*, suggests the possibility that *gufta* migrated from the Red Sea with Indian traders from Bombay to Harar. It most likely spread to Oromo areas from Harar with the introduction of Islam.[61]

Burton (1987, 17) describes the *gufta* of the Harari women in the 1850s:

> The front and back hair parted in the center is gathered in two large bunches below the ears, and covered with dark blue muslin or network, whose ends meet under the chin. This coiffure is bound round the head at the junction of scalp and skin by a black satin ribbon, which varies in breadth according to the wearer's means.

Paulitschke (1888a, 69), in the 1880s tells us: "The women wear their hair back in two balls behind the ear and held together by a fine blue or violet veil called *gufta*. Under the chin the two hair balls are tied with the tassel of the veil."[62] Today, the *gufta* is no longer tied underneath the chin, but fitted back along the hairline.

In Harar, the *gufta* was once made locally on looms by Argobba male weavers for local Argobba, Harari and Oromo women patrons. If the imported *gufta* did come from India, as I suspect, it was copied by Argobba weavers some time during the eighteenth or nineteenth century. One of the last Argobba weavers alive today described the typical loom and the *gufta* production process:

> We made *gufta* by hand on an upright loom called '*shabaakat.*' We prepared the *shabaakat* from a plant called '*gobeensa*' [bamboo]. The loom consists of four pieces of wood made into a rectangle about three feet by two feet. From the wood of *hudha gorbo*[63] we make *qalama*, a needle-like utensil used to finish the edges. Black thread for weaving is purchased from the markets in Harar and Baabile. In two afternoons, I used to produce a completed *gufta*. After *bombei* came, people bought the finished net in the market and I lost business. Today, women sew on colorful dots, called '*ilillii*' and embroider the edges with red thread and a stripe down the center. (B.M.A., March 5, 2000)

The *Gufta* and the *Foota*: Nuptials and Islamic Identity

In Harar, a married woman who can afford it, wears the fashionable *gufta bombei* with *ilillii* either under a scarf in public or uncovered in private. If a woman is sitting in her home, she will allow her shawl to fall from her head and one or both sides of her *gufta* may be exposed. This lax treatment is not practiced, however, outside of her home. Muslim married women who live in or near to urban centers almost always cover their hair when they are away from their compounds in a public place in accordance with Islamic culture.[64] Usually, an imported scarf a few yards in length is tied around the head and a full-length shawl of cotton, rayon or silk called '*foota*' is placed over the head and shoulders so that the upper torso is also concealed. This shared practice among all Muslim women when they enter a public arena is considered an act of religious piety out of respect for Allah, spouses, and male relatives. As one moves further from the Islamic stronghold of towns to rural areas under its jurisdiction where people largely identify as Muslim but do not place as much value in a Qur'anic education and daily prayer, it is not uncommon to see married women, young and old, go around in villages without a head cover. Yet, unless they have just given birth, these women will usually not be without a *gufta*. The *gufta*, regardless of its origins and primacy among other ethnicities, is a metonymic mark for marriage in Oromo thought.[65] More specifically, it signifies that a woman is no longer a virgin. For this reason, an unmarried woman would never wear a *gufta* because she is expected not to be engaging in sexual intercourse.

From the day that her female relatives place the *gufta* on her head, an Oromo woman is usually never without it, except when bathing or redressing or at special moments such as childbirth. By examining the role of the *gufta* and the *foota* side by side, we see the ways in which hair and its supplements become a screen for nuptial and Islamic identity.

As has already been mentioned, the *foota* is most clearly representative of a woman's status as Muslim. With this long cloth she can completely conceal her head and torso, and like her female Muslim neighbors, announce her Islamic belief and the code of conduct associated with it. While this wrapping does cover her hair and shoulders, its placement on the head as a hair cover is not strictly enforced. This notion of the laxity of *foota* wearing is evident in a quote by Richard Burton (1987, 17), who writes in the 1850's: "Women of the upper class, when leaving the house, throw a blue sheet over the head, which, however, is rarely veiled." The *foota* can be removed and readjusted in public and the *gufta* itself may be visible without consequence. For this reason, I am suggesting that the *foota* operates in Oromo belief first and foremost as an external referent of Islamic faith – an outer shell of one's religious conviction. It is neither a permanent fixture nor a necessity to the conception of oneself as Muslim. The *foota* also activates notions of faith and community by connecting Oromo women to their Muslim Harari, Somali, Argobba, and Afar neighbors. The *foota* thereby invokes a sense of Islamic solidarity, especially in cities such as Harar (known locally to be the fourth holiest Islamic city after Mecca, Medina, and Jerusalem and boasting ninety-nine mosques) among married women in civic spaces. When visiting the market, or mosque, asserting one's national and religious identity subsumes the subtler and more secretive ethnic associations during married public life.

The *gufta* obscured beneath the *foota* is, on another level, a very different kind of adornment. As the *gufta* is worn publicly and privately, alone and with others, asleep and awake, it becomes a kind of second skin for a married woman. The black coloring and mesh pattern of the *gufta* even resemble strands of plaited hair. Unlike the *foota* which is meant to invoke a moral code of concealing the hair before man and Allah, the webbing of the *gufta* allows head hair to be visible. The wearing of *gufta* is therefore not about an act of hiding, but rather an act of containing as it relates to ideal womanhood. A married woman is expected to be "contained" in character. This is most clearly articulated through the virtues of patience, restraint, humility, and chastity. Once a woman puts on a *gufta* after marriage, her head hair is no longer cut or braided. Instead, it is allowed to grow long naturally as a woman matures. However, it is not allowed to "stand erect" or fly about while dancing as in adolescence. It becomes a visual indicator of the convention of the wife and mother within marriage and engagement. One explanation for male and female circumcision in African societies is to cut from the male his femaleness (foreskin) and to take from the female her maleness (clitoris). The removal of the clitoris at a young woman's excision among the Afran Qallo is clearly connected to the removal of the prominent *bunti* that "stands erect." The *bunti* is not, however, excised. It is allowed to grow long so that it may lie flat.

The Role of the *Gufta* during the Engagement and Marriage Ceremony

Marriage signals the coupling of a woman's body as a procreative entity to her husband's clan while maintaining blood relations with her own clan through the use of particular dress and hairstyle. While a woman can own property, advance economically, and gain political and social prestige independent from her husband, a wife is considered to belong to his family, and expected to obey any and all restrictions they might place on her. This is also the busiest time of her life. A married woman is responsible for maintaining her household, feeding her family, raising her children, and obligatory labor for her husband's family. She is also likely to have added financial responsibilities. The days of manicured and well-oiled braids are now past, and she simply ties back her loose hair. A song recorded by Paulitschke (1896, 207) laments: "O she, she that has not children. How saturated she is with butter!"[66]

This section probes the manipulation of hair and other key ceremonial objects related significantly to the union of man and wife in the traditional Oromo engagement and wedding ceremony. For marriage to be recognized legally today, an Islamic Shari'a ceremony called '*nikah*' must be performed. The Oromo traditional three-day ceremony usually takes place some weeks prior to the *nikah* but for families who live near Harar there is increasing pressure to conform to Islamic principles and either modify or reduce the elaborate Oromo wedding itself; for example, during the *gudunfa* (engagement ceremony) the act of *hodja* (consuming smoked milk) out of *cicoo* (specially prepared gourds) while discussing the bride price is interspersed with the invocation of the name of Allah and recitations of Qur'anic passages.[67] For this reason, aspects of Oromo traditional engagement and marriage discussed herein come from accounts of ceremonies performed thirty to fifty years ago, and recorded in pastoralist communities in Fedis and Baabile.[68] While these accounts are regionally specific and dated, and may be significantly different than the present ceremony in certain respects, many elements have remained the same, including the hairstyle and hairdressing of the bride, the anointing of the bride and groom with butter, and the exchange of cultural items between the two families. These forms and gestures of the older celebration, including the manipulation of hair, remain important symbols in the abbreviated ceremony today because they act as visual cues to ethical notions of conjugality and gender in the Oromo social structure. In order to investigate hairdressing and the central ideas and objects associated with it, the following section will describe only short segments of the much broader ritual structure of the engagement and marriage ceremonies.

Engagement

Matchmaking may begin between families when children are still infants. If two families decide they would like to betroth their children to each other, the son's parents pay a visit to the daughter's parents. The son's mother brings milk to consume in a *cicoo* tied with *gaadi* (leather rope) and smeared with butter on the vessel's lip. While standing in front of her son's potential in-laws, she ties the *gaadi* and states metaphorically that a woman holding a knife should not sever family relations. Instead, a woman that holds the rope should tie the family together.[69] Later, at their next meeting, the mother of the son carries *siiqee*, a woman's stick cut from the Harooreessa tree. She stands in front of the doorway of the mother of the daughter and announces: "I'm giving a child to you, and I want one from you."[70] If she is in favor of the arrangement, the girl's mother replies: "You shall find what you want and become fat."[71] When the boy's mother is finally invited to sit in the home of the girl's mother, she presents her with the *cicoo* from the first visit. The mothers each drink milk four times from this gourd. Then the girl's mother places her infant daughter in her lap and anoints her forehead and the crown of her head with the *muuduu* (gift butter). The mothers agree that from that day forward they will be in-laws. At the next meeting, another ceremony is performed. This time, the father of the son blesses the union. He likens the marriage of the daughter to the woman's stick, *siiqee* and the marriage of the son to *bordoo*, the thin branch carried by men.[72]

During this three-part exchange between potential in-laws, it is the mothers that first begin the prescribed dialogue for marriage using *ciicoo, gaadi*, and *siiqee*, as symbols of containment and reciprocity, tying and binding, and proper self-government, respectively. The *ciicoo* has been prepared and decorated by the son's mother from milk cows that belong to the *gosa* of the boy – the *gosa* that will someday become the girl's clan if negotiations proceed favorably. It holds the butter and the milk that the boy's mother has prepared. It is also a major household item and suggests the domestic space that the daughter will inhabit in her in-law's village. By tasting these products, the mother of the daughter is said to be sampling the quality of the livestock and, thus, the quality of life that her daughter can expect. The women activate the mixing of their two families through future marriage by sharing this milk. The *gaadi* wound tightly around the gift *ciicoo* reminds the mother of the daughter of the promise of betrothal long after the boy's mother departs. Like the butter, the *gaadi* is also a prepared cattle product of the boy's *gosa*, and the receiver later scrutinizes its preparation quality and strength. The image of the *siiqee and bordoo*, the stick carried by wise women and men who have lived exemplary lives, are conjured up as models of self-discipline for the future bridal pair.

At the end of the first visit, the mother of the girl rubs butter from the gift *ciicoo* onto her daughter's forehead and crown. By dabbing the butter prepared from cows in the possession of the boy's *gosa*, the girl's mother is marking her daughter's destiny (N.A.M., March 18, 2000). The glistening, oily salve is believed to soak into the skin and hair to 'seal the agreement.' The girl's mother will ritually anoint her daughter again publicly during her marriage ceremony but this time with butter from her own cows. In the Islamized regions, the hands and feet of the bride and her attendants are stained red brown with henna paste or the Goshut plant. During the Rako ceremony, a steer is sacrificed, and the betrothed dip their finger in the blood and anoint each other on the breast and genitals. In the past, the bride had her whole body rubbed with blood to ensure pregnancy and the groom poured blood into the depression in her neck to bind her love to him.

Marriage

Fifty years ago, women commonly married around fifteen years of age. Today, they are usually two to five years older. Some 200 years ago under the *gadaa* system, men married in their late thirties or early forties as was accorded their age-grade class. Today, they marry roughly five to ten years younger. Marriage may be delayed due to a young man's lack of resources and his inability to provide a home or a bride price. It is common for young men who cannot afford a bride price to devote a year of service, usually in the form of manual labor, to his future in-laws before the wedding is officiated. Though no longer practiced today, two generations ago it was also possible for young Arsi and Afran Qallo women to choose their husbands in a ceremony called 'Assenna.' During Assenna, a girl of marriageable age who had her eye on a particular boy may enter his family's home early in the morning, scatter grasses and fruit on the floor, and make her intentions known. His family had to honor her request and if, for any reason, the boy could not or would not marry her, his family had to compensate her with livestock.

In most cases, however, marriage is thought of as an arrangement between two families. When a girl child reaches marriageable age, the two families will formally come together again to meet with the Jarsaa Wali Galte, a man who during the time of *gadaa* was the official responsible for overseeing Oromo nuptial law. The boy's family usually brings four cows, called '*meedicha handhuraa*' ('gift' or 'umbilical cord'), and one male goat as a bride price for the girl's family. The Jaarsa Wali Galte examines the cows to his satisfaction, counts them, and orders the goat to be slaughtered. The skin of the front leg of this goat, *meedicha*, is tied on the wrists of the girl and boy. The cows are then given names and they are collectively referred to as '*meedicha handhurra*' ('bellybutton'). The cows stay with the girl's family, but they cannot be sold, traded or slaughtered until the girl marries. Around this same time, the girl's relatives and neighbors present her with *geegayoo* (livestock for her marriage). As these animals are counted by the Jaarsa Wali Galte, the bride's friends sing:

> I plaited your hair; you've become beautiful today. As I churn, I make butter to rub in your hair. Why is your father afraid to let you come out? As I churn, I put braids in your hair. Look, your relatives cannot lose you. Your father divides your cattle from his cattle. And your mother's womb can't feel joy (in losing you).[73]

In this initial wedding gift exchange, the leather of the gift goat is tied at the wrists of the engaged couple, binding them visually to each other through the skin of the same animal. Likewise, the cattle presented to the girl's family serve to unite the two families through a bond as tight as that between a mother and child – the umbilicus. In contrast, the song sung to the young bride by her girlfriends reveals the real-life separation the young woman is about to experience. As the girls sing about the loss that her father and mother will feel, they console her with descriptions of their task to beautify her hair. During this time in her life, the association of her hair with her paternal relatives who have cut, groomed, and styled it throughout her lifetime is very strong. For her wedding and the month afterward, these same girls and women continue to prepare and fuss over her hair, and continue to reassure her by reciting: "Look, your relatives cannot lose you."

At a later ceremony, *gabbara gulanta*, the mother of the bride receives cows from the fiancé's family. The cattle are named collectively '*ijoo haadda*' ('the eye of the mother'). She also receives clothing called '*uwwisa haadda*' (literally, 'cover of the mother). In this case, *ijoo haadda* (the eye of the mother) refers to her daughter (the one who holds her eye) whom she will soon lose. This gift of cattle for the mother acknowledges her loss and offers her, instead, a beautiful animal to catch her eye. The second gift of clothing (cover of the mother) is a gift with which she can metaphorically hide from her loss and cover her sorrow. It is said that in order for this gift to work successfully, the cloth must be beautiful enough to shield a mother's eyes from the absence of her daughter.

Since a daughter's marriage is a heightened emotional state for a mother, the two gifts of cattle and cloth in tandem are intended symbolically to contain her sadness by both distracting and "covering her eyes." In this ritual gift exchange where the mother is placated through beautiful things, the intersection between eye power, object, and containment is concretely expressed. In this engagement ceremony, Oromo women are compensated or "contained" with gifts. The names of both of these gifts make reference to her eyes – a site from which curses or destructive thoughts may be inflicted on others. These older Oromo women are likely post-menopausal, which grants them special status associated with wisdom and discretion within Oromo society, and allows them to participate more fully in male spaces. Informants state that it is the responsibility of the fiancé's parents to "restore harmony to her heart" with gifts so as not to anger the mother (A.S.I., March 11, 2000). If these gifts are not provided, a mother might be overcome with jealousy that could negatively affect the family of the groom.

After *gabbara gulanta,* the mother, accompanied by her friends and relatives, will parade through the village to her home. There her daughter will be waiting to receive them. Her friends will have undone her braids and conditioned her hair with butter. Among the Afran Qallo, at this occasion, her mother makes the first ceremonial part in her hair, dividing it down the middle. This part in the hair symbolizes both the separation that the daughter and her maternal relatives will soon experience and the division that now marks her life – the physical transfer away from her parent's home to the village of her husband. While her blood will remain part and parcel of the *gosa* of her father, her reproductive rights and labor are now under her husband's jurisdiction.

After the mother or another female elder parts her daughter's hair, other female attendants will execute the hair preparation and braid *nanno*. The gift of *manqutt* for her *sabbata* belt, a gift provided by the fiancé during the period of engagement, is now tied around the bride's waist. Among the Wallo, the cloth belt and *amshoo* (blue-black dress) are provided by the mother and the cloth can only be secured at the bride's waist by someone who has never divorced. The bride then sits with her friends. Since she is expected to cry, her friends reinforce the life she is giving up in song in order to emphasize her departure and help bring tears. While she cries, her parents bestow a long list of advice upon her concerning her new role as wife. The last command resonates: "Tie your *sabbata* tight and work hard."[74]

During this exchange, the parents of the bride, with her girlfriends as audience, are symbolically reprimanding their daughter and they do not respond to her tears. This ceremonial event in the home of the daughter's parents is intended to ritually sever her childhood familial ties. Her friends do not console her at this occasion by singing to her as they do during *geegayoo* when the bride receives gift animals. Instead, it is the *sabbata manqutt* that they tie around her waist as she is reminded of her duties. Here the *sabbata* is the central symbol wrapped at her abdomen in much the same way that her hair will be wrapped with a *gufta*. However, while hair comes to stand for her biological *gosa*, the *sabbata* that once tied her thighs during *absuma arabi* connects her to the *gosa* of her husband, who will claim her sex and hence her future children. The binding of her belly with *sabbata* contrasts metaphorically with the opening of her sex through intercourse and childbirth.

During a later ceremony, *guyaa cheeda*, a goat or ox is slaughtered in the village of the groom. Hand in hand, the groom and bride jump over the slaughtered animal and the guests rejoice. For the next day or two, the guests and bridal party enjoy intervals of feasting and dancing. The bride is presented with a new *foota* and in Wallo, *kutaa*, a white textile with color at the hem and cloth for *saddetta* from the groom and his family. Her female and male attendants carry her new clothes so that others may see the quantity and quality of these gifts. During most of her wedding ceremony, the bride wears the iron bracelet *guticha* on her upper arm, the bronze or copper bracelet *kilkillee* at her wrist, *saddetta* made from *mamuudii* cloth, *qarmaa*, and *sakayyoo*, a fragrant plant placed behind the ear. Once she is married and she has begun to live with her husband, she will take off the *mamuudii* cloth and put on *saddetta* made of *abu jedid* cloth. She will also change her waist tie from the predominantly black *manqutt* to the white *durriya*.

During the festivities, the bride and groom spend most of the time either seated in the home of the groom's parents or marching through town, while the wedding guests dance and sing outside the door. Men dance aggressively with sticks, while women dance and drum on *ghee* cans, praising the groom and his clan by singing: "*Oromo eey da*" ("He is an Oromo, we are proud of being Oromo"). When the bride emerges from the house wrapped in her white *saddetta*, she carries her *siiqee* stick with her. The groom holds a whip and a knife. He wears a white, long-sleeved shirt and a white textile wrapped around his waist. As the bride and groom proceed through the village with their attendants, old women who meet them on the road may bless the party by anointing them with butter on their forehead and the big toe of their right foot. The bride and groom are anointed again by the bride's mother with butter from her cows. As she dabs the butter on their forehead and hair, she reminds them that while her daughter's body is now in the care of her new husband, her daughter's blood still belongs to her father's *gosa*.

Later, the parents of both bride and groom bless the couple in front of their new home with their aspersion, called *tufta*, which involves the spraying of saliva on the head by pursing the lips, placing the tongue close to the lips and administering an "s" sound. *Tufta* is a common form of blessing from elders to the youth. At marriage, it has particular significance for the bride and her mother. When asked why the mother spits on the forehead and hair of her daughter, three common answers were given. First, she is thought to be instilling a blessing for her daughter and her son-in-law. Second, she is expelling the saliva of her biological family to affix her daughter to her blood relations. Third, before spitting, mothers will call out: "I am praying to you from my womb" and since salivary fluid is thought to exist in the mouth, throat, and belly, she passes liquid from her womb to her daughter as symbolic procreation. In this sense, the procreative potential of the fertile stomach fluid of the mother that nurtured the daughter when she was a fetus should be passed to the child of the daughter.

The Placement of the *Gufta* after *Arooza*

After the marriage ceremony, the bride and groom enter into *arooza* – the month of leisure. During *arooza*, the bride and groom receive gifts, food, and blessings from visiting neighbors, and they are entertained by their friends in the groom's parents' home. In the evenings, the women dance *hellee* and the men and women dance *shuguyyee*. When drinking milk, the bride and groom share the same cup, symbolically binding them to the animals that will become their livelihood. After this period of inactivity where no work is required from either of them, the bride returns to her mother's home.

The next few weeks in her mother's village are called '*weedu*' and they are considered her last weeks as a member of her childhood *gosa*. During this month, she must go to the river to wash clothes with her friends to signify that she has established her own household and she will oversee and perform her duties correctly. On the occasion of washing, she takes with her two gourds that belong to her mother's household. One she uses to aid her in clothes washing, while the other is thrown into the current of the river. The gourd that floats away represents the first *cicoo* that her mother was given by her husband's mother when her daughter was only a baby. The new bride also learns the proper preparation for *biddena* (traditional bread) and she sings praises to her family members who have died. During *weedu*, her mother prepares the essentials for her daughter's *alaa tattu* (new home), which she will carry back with her at the end of her stay.

For these first two months of marriage, a new wife does not wear the *hamasha*, *nassii* or *gufta*. These hairdressings are reserved for the end of *weedu* when the time has come for her to return to her husband's village. At her departure, her mother and her female relatives place a stool outside of her mother's home. The daughter sits facing the direction of her husband's village while her female relatives undo her braids. The women create *hamasha*, the hairstyle in which the hair is divided down the center and tied together at the nape in two billowing balls. In the meantime, the *gufta* is soaked in a bowl with milk, tree sap, and tree resin. When the hairstyle is complete and the *gufta* is ready to be placed on her head, only those women who themselves have living parents, a living husband, and children participate. They put the *gufta* on the bride and sing to her.

When they have finished tying the *gufta* and securing it with *shaashii* or *nassii*, the bride begins the journey back to her husband's village with the help of her friends. In the meantime, the groom has spent the month with his family. They too have been busy with *wadaajaa* (performing prayer ceremonies) and *kismidal* (making food offerings). On the day that the groom is to return to his new home, his father cuts a tree branch to give to his son to symbolize his new role. The father blesses his son and prays: "Let the bride become the mother of the house and wear her *gufta*, and let the groom become the father and take this stick."

During this period of separation, the bride goes through a series of symbolic acts (many more than what are mentioned here) that clearly mark her separation from her parents and emphasize her new role. In particular, the manipulation of her hair serves as a tangible, external sign of her new status, as well as a more personal, internal reference to her familial heritage and its expectations. Certainly, the *hamasha* style and the *gufta* on her head alert others to her status as a wife in the village of her husband. However, the fact that the *hamasha* is formed by the hands of female relatives and the fact that the *gufta* is soaked in milk from the cows of her *gosa,* creates for the bride a feeling of solidarity with her kin that helps her through the difficulties to come (K.U., February 15, 2000).

In contrast, owing to the strong affiliation hair holds with a woman's mother and her paternal relations, the *gufta* acts as kind of screen that separates a bride from her adolescent ties. When her husband's parents pray for proper marriage at the end of *weedu,* they conjure up the image of the suitable wife as a woman who wears *gufta.* The *gufta* itself can visually stand for a married woman. In this manner, the placement of the *gufta* on the bride superimposes a new identity onto an older one. Furthermore, the *gufta* operates as a container for the unbraided hair, keeping it flat, manageable, and "unwild."

One anomaly, of course, are the two balls created through the *hamasha* hairstyle that billow out at the nape of the neck (Figure 6.18). These rounded forms could be characterized as symbols of fertility due to their breast-like shape or they could suggest the fullness of pregnancy. However, neither of these visual equivalences was suggested either in discussions with women or in the ritual context. What was mentioned, however, was the way in which the *gufta* denotes time (S.Y., February 14, 2000). When women age, their hair loses its fullness and their *hamasha* balls begin to droop. In much the same way breasts sag and flatten with gravitational pull over a lifetime, the hair also thins and transforms. The height at which the *gufta* falls, which may range from just below the line of the ear to below the shoulders, and the plumpness of the ball itself, mirror a married woman's aging process.

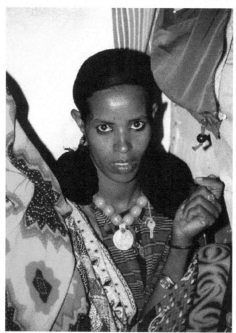

Figure 6.18 A Married Afran Qallo Woman wearing the Hamasha Hairstyle with Facial Tumtuu

There are just two occasions when a woman removes her *gufta* and her hair is allowed to remain unprepared for forty days: (1) following childbirth and (2) after the death of her husband. Both are occasions that signal a dangerous period through the rejection of bodily norms. Hair is not dressed during *gufufa* (mourning) for either the death of a husband or, in some cases, the death of a child or other close relative. Traditionally, an Oromo woman removes her jewelry and wears the same clothes that she had on when her husband died for four months and fifteen days. She washes only once a week, does not enter a mosque, and does not comb or butter her uncovered hair.

Childbirth

When a woman is ready to give birth to her first child, she sends for her mother. Her mother brings her a leather mat prepared from *ijoo haadda,* one of the original heifers she received at her daughter's marriage. This mat is intended to catch her daughter's blood and make labor more comfortable. After birth, a woman stays in the confines of her home with her newborn for a period of forty days. While women close to her will visit and provide for her, she does not receive other callers, as she is considered to be both physically weary, and vulnerable to human and spiritual harm. During this liminal period, both mother and child are thought to be particularly susceptible to negative spiritual forces. To protect herself before birth in the past, a mother close to eight months pregnant called her married female friends and they performed *daraayaa*, an Afran Qallo version of the *atete* ceremony in which fertility is celebrated. The women brought *cicoo*, *gaadi*, and *siqqee*, and they prepared *marqaa* porridge, drank *hodja*, and sung blessings for the mother and child. They asked the female deity *Atete* to shield the mother and child from bad things, and they prayed that the baby be released peacefully.

Paulitschke records a festival among the Afran Qallo Oromo and those residing south of Shoa that parallels the memories of my informants, whereby the expectant mother has her hair colored white or grey at her temples to identify her condition. This happens when she first learns that she is pregnant. The ceremony includes drumming, singing, and gift-giving. The colored hair is later cut off with scissors and, from this moment on, the pregnant woman lets her hair down and gives up heavy work. When she is ready to deliver, a midwife assists her. She drinks a strong concoction made from the bark and leaves of the acacia shrub, and births while squatting. An amulet is placed on her neck just before the baby crowns. Once the child is born, her friends wash her, nourish her with butter, myrrh, and smoke, and help her breastfeed. When the umbilical cord falls off, it might be placed on the door of the home or tied to the neck of a horse or cow that has been gifted to the child. The child will take his or her name from the individual who gave the animal that now wears its umbilicus. The elders come to bless the child. Spirits are also called for the well-being of the baby for which the parents must provide a sacrifice.

A new mother signals her physical state and combats maleficent mystical intentions by removing her jewelry, except among Arsi women, who put on the barrel-shaped metal forehead ornament, *qanafa* (Figure 4.3). The *qanafa*, worn four to five months after birth, signals that a woman is in *wayyuu* (a liminal, sacred state) (Østebø 2009, 1051). It also indicates her exclusion from hard labor and sexual activity. During post-labor, a new mother does not cut her nails or comb, wash or dress her hair. Unkempt hair that is neither pleasantly fragrant nor visually attractive is said to repel negative spiritual forces and the advances of husbands. She may wash her body, but she avoids soap and sits naked periodically over burning incense. This incense bath, called '*ulacuu*,' is also intended to keep *jarri* and *jinn* at bay by engulfing her body and the entrance to her womb with smoke.

To protect her child who is also considered to be quite vulnerable for the first month after birth, she keeps knives and other metal implements near her sleeping mat to drive away or distract harmful spirits who have come to examine the newborn.[75] Among the Wallo, the baby may even be given the water to drink with which the knife has been washed. *Jinn* are believed to be responsible for startling newborns from their sleep and causing their little bodies to jolt when they are awake. For this reason, incense is also continually burned near the infant and a piece of *qumbii* (strong-smelling resin) is tied to the infant's wrist. Once the child reaches his or her fourth month, this resin bracelet is replaced with a string of blue glass beads called '*doqa*.'

After forty days, the baby is brought forth from the home, given a name, and introduced to the community. The same day the mother returns to her home to wash and comb her hair, make *hamasha*, reposition her *gufta*, and resume normal activity. In the previous discussion of marriage, *gufta* became a metaphor for self-containment, while wild, teased hair became a metaphor for warriorhood and aggression. To combat the susceptibility to illness and supernatural harm during childbirth and the weeks that follow, women draw on the strength of their exposed, unkempt hair. This hair acts as guardian to the potential threats posed by a husband, spirits or other humans until a mother regains her strength.

The manipulation of hair from a natural state to that which is socially prescribed and meaningful resonated within all life stages of an Oromo woman; for example, new growth of hair on a previously exposed scalp communicates the end of childhood. A married woman screens in and contains her hair in a hairnet to signal a shift in affiliation and reproductive rights from that of her parent's clan to that of her husbands. Old age and the sagging breasts that accompany it resonate in the elongated and withered balls of her *gufta*.

The Oromo, like many other societies, have crafted their hair to reflect their aesthetic and moral ideals during various cycles of life. While some discrepancy existed in the past between agricultural and pastoral head dressings, and the complete shaving of the head at excision is no longer practiced, the adoption of specific hairstyles and hairdressings at significant moments in the lifecycle has endured. Even as lifecycle rituals are amended to adopt Islamic elements or objects are altered to distinguish new fashions, hair, as a fluctuating, moldable medium itself, remains the central element in lifecycle rituals.

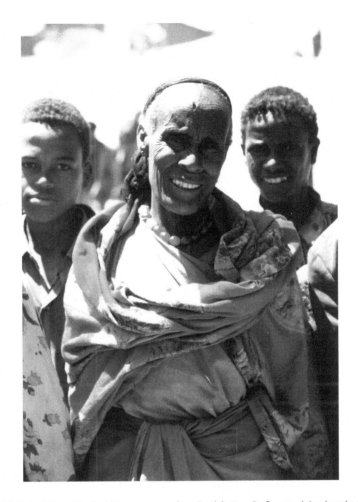

Figure 6.19 Elderly Afran Qallo Woman wearing Saddetta, Gufta and Amber in Kombolcha

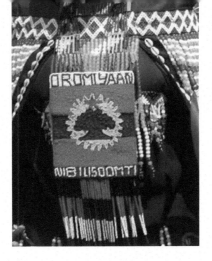

Chapter Seven:

Blending the Old with the New

On-going Issues of Identity and Dress in the Emergence of Oromo Nationalism

In the previous discussion of hair as an extension of the body, and the ways that hair is manipulated and adorned during a woman's lifecycle, no clear conceptual distinctions were drawn between hair and hair decorations. Hair in its length, shape, and style, and hairdressing as a means of drawing attention to, or away from, the hair, mark the formalized and celebrated moments of an Oromo woman's life. Both function as non-verbal communicators of issues surrounding marriage, morality, and womanhood. This blurring of body parts and body art in earlier discussions of Oromo folklore, traditional judiciary practices, and spirit beliefs, too, is part and parcel of the Oromo aesthetic classification. Objects must be activated on the body for efficacy or, as one Nole elder mentioned: "They need each other to work" (K.U., February 28, 2016). Further, as new situations arise, new ways of adorning and framing the self are invoked.

Among the Barentuma Oromo, a series of codes shaped through a shared past, common religious belief, and conditions of subordination dictate bodily restraints, and determine which collective physical representations are withheld or reproduced at particular moments and within specific contexts. In this chapter, we find that the growing Oromo nationalist movement informed first by conditions of subordination within the Ethiopian state and, as of this writing, hope and disappointment in the newly elected Prime Minister Dr. Abiy Ahmed, is activated in new dress types. The cultural glue of this nationalist movement within Oromia and the Oromo Diaspora is largely founded on the shared experience of language, history, and political domination. The *gadaa* or *raba-dori* system and, to a minor extent, women's *siqqee* institutions, common to all Oromo, are often promoted as a socio-political organizing ideology through which to mold an independent Oromo nation.[76] While both Oromo men and Oromo women throughout Oromia can lay claim to this shared experience, including the move from the stratified grades of the *gadaa* institution to the court system enforced by the Ethiopian state, the loss of rights to grazing and farm lands, and increased state-sponsored violence, Oromo nationalism has been most publicly formulated and articulated by educated Oromo men in a male-centered paradigm. Kuwee Kumsa (1998, 155) reports that Oromo national movements, particularly the Oromo Liberation Front, have not adequately acknowledged the role of women in its struggle and its formation nor has the organization included a women's voice. Further, the placement of women and dress has only recently been formally acknowledged as a relevant component of nationalist sentiment.

Yet, in my discussions surrounding nationalism and dress within Oromo communities, women's bodies and their personal arts were viewed as instrumental in the projection, albeit subtle and symbolic, of Oromo identity and Oromo consciousness. Further, women were viewed as the dominant creators and transmitters of Oromo cultural symbols. The reason the decorated female body is left out of this debate has much to do with the ways in which Oromo nationalism was first conceptualized as an abstract ideal among urban, educated men. The establishment of the Macha-Tuluma self-help organization among the Oromo in the 1963 and the participation in government sponsored programs under the military Derg regime (1974–1991), coupled with an increased exposure to secondary education and urban jobs, created a uniquely modern Oromo consciousness for young men (H. Lewis 1996, 43). As Mekuria Bulcha (1996, 49) has written: "The role of articulating, defining and promoting Oromo identity was assumed by a fledgling intelligentsia beginning in the mid-1960s." In this male-centered political climate, the expressions of rural women in localized areas went largely unnoticed. However, women in this period were independently creating a material expression of the emerging nationalism sweeping the Oromo countryside (J.A., February 3, 2000).

After an overview of Oromo nationalist ideology and its birth within the Ethiopian state, this chapter will focus on three kinds of dress: (1) a modern, machine-made dress or skirt, (2) a beaded necklace, and (3) facial markings.

Nationalism and Body Ideology

In his classic study of nationalism, E. J. Hobsbawn (1990, 9, 10) draws out a notion of nationhood that belongs "exclusively to a particular, and historically recent, period . . . situated at the point of intersection of politics, technology and social transformation" and is further "constructed essentially from above." In a similar light, Gellner (quoted in Vale 1992, 54) defines 'nationalism' as "the consequences of a new form of social organization, based on deeply internalized education-dependent high cultures each protected by the state."

The emergence of an Oromo identity, which is both born from ethnic affiliation and informed by it, was not originally imagined by only a technologically sophisticated and well-educated elite nor was it protected by the state. Oromo nationalism essentially contradicts the definitions proposed by Hobsbawn and Gellner. The sense of Oromummaa has strong connections to the past and is actively discussed as easily in student dormitories as cattle markets. The emergence of Oromo nationalism has been linked to the 1960s and 1970s as a response to unequal economic and political representation, the experiences of colonization, feudalism, imperial rule, and state-sponsored violence against the Oromo throughout the past century. It is as much an ethnic construct as a nationalist one, since Oromo nationalism has continued to be reformulated among the Oromo on a local (ethnonational), state (national), and international (pan-Oromo) level.

As discussed earlier, the crucial time at the turn of the twentieth century when all Oromo were incorporated into the Ethiopian empire by Menelik II led to the demise of the most central Oromo institutions. Owing to the unique experiences of the Afran Qallo under the rule of the Harari emirs and Egyptian forces prior to the arrival of Menelik II, these institutions had already been in decline for a quarter of a century. By the first reign of Haile Selassie (1916–1936), the Ethiopian state officially refused to acknowledge ethnic diversity in order to unify the country and promote the Amharic language, religion, and culture of the ruling Amhara elite.[77] Yet the creation of an Ethiopian nationalism was never fully realized due to competing nationalisms among its varied cultures.

After the Italian Occupation (1936–1941), which largely supported Oromo cultural and judicial practices and religion, Haile Selassie tried again to create national unity by dissolving the positions of the traditional monarchic leaders, abolishing the Gabbar serf system, and centralizing the government. However, he did not pave the way toward emancipation for the peoples of Ethiopia nor did he allow oppressed ethnicities into prominent governmental or military positions reserved for his newly created bureaucratic–military bourgeoisie. He agreed to join Eritrea in a federation as dictated by the United Nations but soon thereafter he used aggression to annex Eritrea in 1962 while the United Nations looked the other way. As I. M. Lewis (1983, 4) states: "[T]his represented a signal victory for centralist Amhara nationalism. The dynastic rule continued with new territory and Western support."

While political parties were outlawed, disgruntled students and teachers, civil servants, and military members began organizing secretly to dislodge Haile Selassie's government. The benefits of nationalized education and the mass media allowed peoples in isolated areas to understand their situations more fully, and band together to contemplate means for action. There followed a failed military coup (1960), the Bale Oromo peasant resistance (1963–1970), and the formation of the Eritrean People's Liberation Front (EPLF), the Tigray People's Liberation Front (TPLF) and the OLF. In 1974, Emperor Haile Selassie and his government were deposed, and a socialist-inspired provisional government called the 'Derg' (Amharic for 'Committee') emerged, dominated by Colonel Mengistu Haile Maryam.

Hoping to secure self-determination after years of exploitation, Eritrean and Somali nationalists immediately asked for secession but were met with complete resistance, including the mobilization of Operation Red Star in 1982, which tried to seize Eritrean land under the Ethiopian flag. Mengistu had "adopted what his opponents regard as an extreme form of Amhara chauvinist nationalism" (I. M. Lewis 1983, 8). Mengistu sought to socialize the country by enforcing loyalties to the state and not to what he perceived as ethnocentricity (Triulzi 1983, 112). As Triulzi mentions: "All attempts at individual solutions, involving separate struggles, were seen therefore as dangerous since they might undermine the effort to bring about a unified national struggle" (112). As Mengistu's regime became more brutal, people's hopes for emancipation and long-delayed democratic reforms slipped away.

After a long struggle, the EPLF, the TPLF, and OLF defeated the military regime in May 1991. The EPLF opted for an independent Eritrea, while the TPLF and the OLF formed the Transitional Government of Ethiopia (1991–1992). However, in June 1992, conflict broke between the TPLF and the OLF. The more powerful TPLF, militarily defeated the OLF and banned that organization. The TPLF created the EPRDF, through which that organization dominated Ethiopian political landscape from 1992 to 2018. Jalata (1998, 14) writes that the Tigrayan liberation movement was "mainly interested in taking power from the Amhara rulers and keeping the Ethiopian empire under their control by introducing cosmetic changes." In contrast, the OLF fought for the total transformation of the Ethiopian Empire. Even after the establishment of nine regional states, including Oromia – the Oromo regional state – the people were not allowed to administer themselves freely, as the TPLF security officials tightly controlled Oromia.

While the main body of literature devoted to Ethiopian studies continues to focus on Highland Christian Ethiopia's history, a recent surge in scholarship is drawing attention to these issues, and to the Oromo and other traditionally subordinated peoples. The great feats learned by all schoolchildren of the famous exploits of Emperor Yohannis IV (1872–1889), who united the historical Abyssinian kingdom in northern Ethiopia, and Emperor Menelik II (1889–1913), who created the modern Ethiopian Empire, and defeated the Italian imperial forces at the Battle of Adowa in 1896, are being rewritten as images of Amhara colonization by historians and anthropologists sympathetic to the voices of the periphery.

The experience of the Oromo in Ethiopia has been characterized in this literature as a colonizing experience.[78] Jalata (1998, 27) expresses emerging Oromo nationalism as "a program of national liberation" grounded in "the common experience of colonial oppression." In the popular imagination, however, the image of Ethiopia has provided the West and non-Western alike with a common model of an African monarchy that resisted colonization by Western powers. "However discriminatory and harsh the Amhara hegemony might be in its treatment of subjected populations inside the country, to the outside world and specially the under-privileged of the third world, Ethiopia offered a resplendent symbol of Black Power" (I. M. Lewis 1983, 4). When Ghana gained independence in 1957, Nkrumah and his council modeled the new Ghanaian flag, with the red and yellow, on the red stripes of the Ethiopian flag to create a pan-African symbol. Further, Rastafarianism, especially in the Caribbean world, advocates Ethiopia as the biblical center of African civilization, and the symbol of unity and strength against the colonial monster. Ethiopia as a country free from Western political domination became for the black African Diaspora an image of hope and freedom. During the time of the Italian Occupation, for example, displaced Africans the world over organized public protests and tried to enlist in the Ethiopian army. The pan-Africanist Edward William Blyden (quoted in Robinson 1985, 60) referred to the Ethiopian heritage as "the most creditable of ancient peoples" and claimed that they had achieved "the highest rank of knowledge and civilization."

Odaa, the Sycamore Tree

There is obviously much work to be done to dispel the notion of Ethiopia as an ancient, homogenized Christian kingdom that resisted Western colonization. Even more so, awareness of the Oromo and other marginalized groups, and their current situation within the Ethiopian state is vital. The most powerful force today is social media. The first half of 2016 saw an increase in state-sponsored violence, including the killing of over 400 mostly young Oromo, political intimidation, and gross human rights violations. Months before, Oromo farmers and herders near the town of Ginchi west of the capital learned that they would be forcibly removed from their fertile farming and forest lands. When people learned of the federal government's plan to parcel out millions of hectares of land in Oromia to foreign investors and large-scale industry, and to expand the area of the capital, Addis Ababa, into Oromia state (Addis Ababa Integrated Development Master Plan), they began to mobilize in protest. The security forces responded with lethal force. Owing to the lack of independent media in Ethiopia and trustworthy coverage, Oromo in Oromia and the Diaspora took to social media to alert the international community, and to conduct and document protests in major cities across the globe. Facebook and other social media sources erupted with images of men and women in demonstration, bodies lying in the street, and music videos produced around these events. In the videos, Oromo bodies are draped in white garments emblazoned with the *odaa* (sycamore) tree holding the Oromo flag and women are featured with beaded headband (Holcomb and Klemm 2018). The *gadaa* chafe assembly, and all major rituals and political activities were once held under the shade of the *odaa* tree – it is a nationally recognized marker of sacrality, democracy, and Oromo land. Today, the unisex symbols of *odaa*, the Oromo flag, and women's beaded headbands have become key markers of a pan-Oromo identity in the resistance struggle against the government. The national banner or flag of the OLF carries an emblem of the *odaa* tree framed by a yellow star, symbolizing the democracy of the nation. Owning or displaying this flag or clothing made with the image of the OLF flag was illegal in Oromia until 2018 (Figure 7.1). At the time of this writing, *odaa* symbolism has made its way into local and transnational dress styles in permanent and meaningful ways (Figure 7.2).

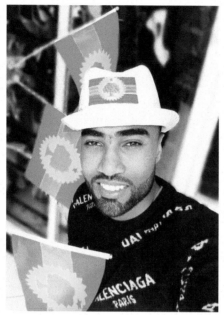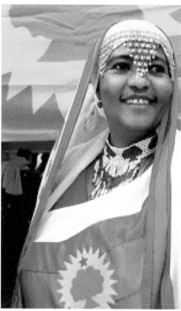

Figure 7.1 The Symbol of Odaa on the Oromo Flag, a Hat and a Beaded Necklace (Left Photograph: Courtesy of Yasin Ib, Right Photograph: Courtesy of Tunsia Mohammed)

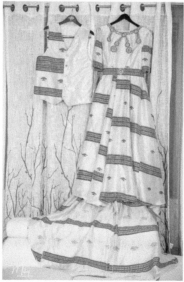

Figure 7.2 Oromo Wedding Dress and Groom's Vest with Odaa (Photograph: Courtesy of Mickey Photography)

In the previous chapters, dress has been organized within the domains of aesthetics and morality, gender and cosmology, and the tensions inherent in aesthetic value, that is, inviting versus hiding, binding versus opening, beautifying versus disfiguring. Included in this polarized structuring of dress is also its ability to include and exclude. As Barnes and Eicher (1992, 1) write: "[D]ress serves as a sign that the individual belongs to a certain group, but simultaneously differentiates the same individual from all others." This book has focused largely on the collective, commemorative statements of dress as they relate to and translate Oromo historical memory. The following section introduces three types of contemporary body art invented in the early 2000s by the Afran Qallo: (1) *mashiinii* (a colorful dress), (2) *ambarka* (a type of beaded necklace), and (3) *kula* (the application of pigment to the face). These art forms are recent transformations of older body art styles. They impart subtle cues about what it means to be Afran Qallo today, at times of uncertainly when being Oromo is dangerous, and at times of hope as they enter into deeper allegiances with the international community.

The Transition of the Dress *Saddetta*

The dress of white sheeting, *saddetta*, is still the dominant dress style among rural women, particularly post-menopausal women who have not married into Somali families or settled in Somali-dominated communities where a *gu'aa* (plaid cloth wrapper) and a *durriyya* (print cloth tunic) are more popular. However, more and more, the pressures of Islam to keep shoulders concealed have resulted in a layering of the upper torso with polyester T-shirts, silk wraps or imported gauzes. In most cases, the *saddetta* remains intact, tied beneath the T-shirt, but among young girls the torso cloth is allowed to hang free and the *saddetta* becomes merely a skirt. In addition, a modern version of the *saddetta*, called '*mashiinii*,' named after the sewing machine, used in its creation, became popular in the last generation.

When not being worn, the *saddetta* is first gathered into inch-long pleats by two women holding each end, then twisted and knotted to keep the pleats in place, and, finally, stored as a tight ball. This creates pressed folds in the material for the next wear. Similarly, the modern *mashiinii* skirt is sewn into permanent pleats to mimic the accordion folds created by hand in *abu jedid* or *mamuudi* cloth.

In the case of the *mashiinii* dress, we find that techniques and materials sometimes less than a decade old have become the fashion of choice among younger generations of Afran Qallo women. The *mashiinii* dress is sewn from imported rayon–cotton blends with brightly colored patterns into a tailored bodice and a full skirt (Figure 7.3). This *mashiinii* dress style allows women to wear the latest prints that make their way into the market, while maintaining the main visual cues of the *saddetta*. Most *mashiinii* cloth is manufactured in Asia and transported via the Red Sea overland from ports in Djibouti to Harar's Taiwan Market, a burgeoning shopping area named after the place from which many of its manufactured items originate. Women can choose from a dozen or so patterned textiles found in Taiwan's makeshift stalls and commission a male tailor to sew the dress with its laborious accordion pleats. Skilled Harari tailors in Taiwan have already internalized Oromo tastes and begun to create readymade *mashiinii* to be taken to local villages. While *mashiinii* is fashionable and worn by women throughout northeastern Oromia in place of *saddetta*, the essence of the Oromo dress is still preserved in the creased pleats of the skirt.

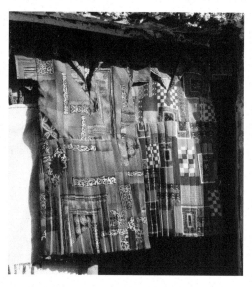

Figure 7.3 The Mashiinii Dress sewn from Imported Prints

I have argued that the *saddetta* as a turn-of-the-century transformation of the indigenous Oromo leather garment is historically rich. The *mashiinii* is certainly embedded in this tradition. As a modern dress, however, it also carries with it a modern structure and a contemporary grammar that resonates in discussions of Oromo consciousness. Once, while I was interviewing a woman about her experiences during the Marxist regime, she repeatedly traced the folds of the pleats in her skirt. Explaining how she and her family had endured several years in prison and several more years in hiding, she pointed at the cloth to suggest the movement to and from detention centers, the periods of seclusion in the forest, and in the homes of relatives: "Here is where we hide" (K.A.M., April 12, 2000). The permanently rendered folds of cloth functioned for her as a visual metaphor of the thematic bookends that run throughout this research – hiding versus being visible. Tangibly embedded in the pleats of the *saddetta* and the *mashiinii* is the suggested interplay of concealment and revelation as it relates to violence, politics, and persecution.

Ambarka Beaded Necklace

The second aspect of dress relevant to a discussion of contemporary Afran Qallo identity is the beaded necklaces called '*ambarka*' (Figure 7.4). The *ambarka* is regularly worn by young women in areas east and south of Harar by the Alla and Baabile. Slight variations in *ambarka* design are also worn in other Afran Qallo areas but they have different names. Among the Jarso, the beaded necklaces are called '*challee*' ('the beads of *atete*'), and among the Nole and Alla, the necklaces are known as '*qudhaaba*' ('ten'). *Ambarka* is constructed either of two thick, single beaded bands joined at the bottom in a series of beaded rows that end with vertically oriented, fringed beaded strands or two double beaded bands connected at the bottom and fringed. In both cases, the sides of the necklace rest flat on the chest, one-and-a-half to three inches in diameter, reaching from the breastbone to the collarbone of a young woman.

The young women who make these necklaces bead imported seed beads onto twine in diamond-shaped patterns framed within broad registers of a single color. The unused twine at the top is further braided into two strands to secure the *ambarka* at the neck. These seed beads from the Czech Republic are purchased in single-color strands sold in abundance since 1990 in the markets of Harar, Fedis, and Baabile, and most readily available in white, green, yellow, blue, and red.

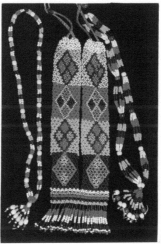

Figure 7.4 (Center) Ambarka Beaded Necklace with (Left and Right) Two Thin Beaded Necklaces

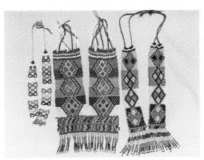

(Center and Right) Two Ambarka Necklaces with (Left) Challee Qarma

Ambarka, along with the beaded headbands, *bishanni* and *challee qarmaa*, make up a complete set of torso adornment (Figure 7.5). These items are most commonly worn together by unmarried girls who are taught to bead in seclusion and who wear only those beaded items they themselves have assembled. Young women pride themselves on never creating the same pattern twice. For this reason, beadwork provides a relatively recent avenue for personal creativity. Women who can afford the spectrum of bead colors can create a variety of looks, as long as they follow the prescribed stylistic code. This code requires a series of diamond shapes dissected by two diagonal lines situated within a sequence of horizontal bands. Beaders may vary the thickness, number of the bands and diamonds, and color in each necklace to create variety.

It may at first appear odd that necklaces only a decade old would possess such rigid stylistic conventions. However, these necklaces are actually very close in style and production to a long-standing tradition of basket making (Figure 7.6). Woven fiber baskets were used until recently in almost every household activity and they served as the main decoration in the home. While baskets still play a role as household containers and they make up part of a woman's dowry, the laborious task of fine basket making is practiced less and less.

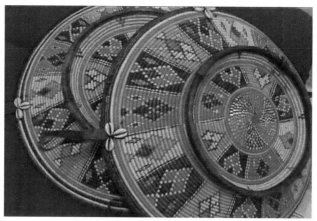

Figure 7.6 Oromo Baskets

As is true throughout Africa, the introduction of imported tin platters, cast-iron cooking pots, and plastic dishes and buckets in the last fifty years has slowed the production of pottery and basketry. Afran Qallo women have largely given up the personal control they once had in producing their own household and ceremonial wares. What a woman uses in her home is now dictated by her financial resources and an aesthetic of foreign manufactured goods.

The reason for this is partly due to the cement walls that are currently replacing regional thatch or mud walls which are not suited to display hand-made baskets or even modern metal stenciled platters. Women also state that the major famines since the 1980s, coupled with the current political climate, have created situations for migration and displacement among the Afran Qallo. Women do not pass the time preparing beautiful houses and decorating the walls with painted designs as they once did in the past, and notions of home are no longer rooted geographically. Instead, the previous creative energy spent in the decoration of interior spaces is now focused on the production of body art. Women hang beautifully patterned bead necklaces on themselves just as they once placed baskets on the walls of their homes (Figure 7.6). If expressions of an Afran Qallo identity were ever located in symbols other than the body, this consciousness is today emerging through the frame of the self.

While beaded sets embody a woman's personal statement, I would argue that they also serve as a medium through which she can display a subverted political voice. The recent change in material in young women's headbands from *qarmaa loti* to *bishanni* and the introduction of *ambarka* in the last ten years can be viewed as a political move by Oromo women to create distance from their Harari neighbors with whom they have had growing political tensions over land and demographic representation by designing new forms that bear no resemblance to Harari ornament. Secondly, Oromo women describe the strands of the favored beads that flood the market as progressive and worldly. They point out that women all over Africa wear jewelry made of these beads and even visitors from outside Africa seem to want them. Thus, women use these new plastic and glass beads from India, China, and the Czech Republic to create global allegiances to notions of Africa and the world beyond. A necklace is also one ornament shared by all divisions of the great Oromo confederacy throughout Ethiopia, Somalia, and Kenya (though materials and form vary widely). While women infrequently travel great distances, they express a desire to want to connect with other Oromo groups that make up the millions of Oromo population outside their own Afran Qallo lineages. Distinguishing themselves through beadwork is one way to create visual participation in emerging Oromo nationalism as young, unmarried women.

The stylistic choices of diamonds and horizontal bands are also significant in this discussion of nationalism and Oromo identity. Certainly, women are drawing on basketry as a model in their beading of the *ambarka* through the same concerns with containment of shapes, the repetition of form and pattern, primary color sets, and the use of stripes and diamonds. We know from Paulitschke (1896, 162) that 120 years ago, the rhombus was the most reproduced figure in dress and jewelry designs, and on the flat expanses of everyday objects.[79] Yet, if we review the *ambarka*, we notice that the *ambarka* diamonds are further divided by two differently colored diagonals. When I asked what this division of the diamond was called, women told me that it was simply known as 'Afran Qallo.' At first, the divided diamond appeared to me to merely serve as an Afran Qallo signature that expressed a woman's beading skill. In hindsight, I believe that there is more to it. This divided diamond pattern is unique to the *ambarka* and is a recent beading pattern. It emerged at the end of a very brutal regime at a time when the government had forbidden the writing of the Oromo language, the speaking of the Oromo language in school, and all forms of Oromo nationalism. In this context, this divided diamond pattern may directly represent the Afran Qallo or, more specifically, "the four sons of Qallo." The larger diamond is

Afran Qallo and the four smaller diamonds are his four sons from which all Afran Qallo trace their genealogy: Alla, Obborra, Baabile, and Daga.

Kula Facial Markings

Throw up your head in the air, tilt it
and lay your *naannoo*[80] in harmony
Shaggee of straight nose[81]
Black-edged eyelids and close eyebrows
that look as if they are carved
"your *kula*[82] and *qarmaa*[83]
faroora[84] and *kulkultaa*[85]
I saw, they look as if they are flawlessly created."
(Lines from the song "Mari Mee," recorded in 1994)

In the song "Mari Mee," above, the singer compliments the decorated space between the young woman's eyes. As has already been elaborated, this area is a central focus for cosmetics. Adorning the face with colored pigment known as '*kula*' was first implemented through tattooing in conjunction with scarification. Today, there is shift away from tattooing to a commodified item of fashion: nail polish. Today, nail polish is applied to the bridge of the nose, between the eyebrows, and to the cheeks (Figure 7.7). Nail polish decoration, which exists side by side with *tumtuu* (tattooing), and *haaxixa* (scarification), falls along a continuum in the indigenous practice of facial alteration.

Scars placed above the eyebrow, along the bridge of the nose, and on the cheeks are intended to heal, protect, and beautify. The process of scarification and tattooing is usually discussed as a feature-enhancing cosmetic today that, such as dots of polish, adds to a woman's attractiveness. However, marks around the eyes are also meant to divert the gaze of strangers who could potentially inflict harm through attack with the evil eye. Nail polish operates both within this belief system as a way of diverting the gaze from the eye area but also as a beautifying agent intended to harness visual attention. Adorning the body to invite the attention of mates or to hide from those with *buda* speaks to issues of disclosure and concealment inherent in all cosmetics used by Oromo women.

Women say they like nail polish for its impermanence, its color variety, and its foreign manufacture. While permanent scars and tattoos bleed, fade, and shift over time, nail polish can be applied quickly and painlessly, then scraped off and reapplied. Even though *kula* made with polish is becoming increasingly popular, the practices of scarring and tattooing persist.[86] The continuation of these processes suggests their significance as cultural codes that largely resist the ongoing changes associated with fashion.

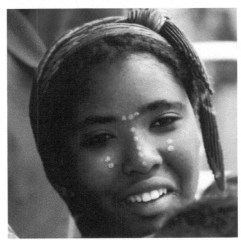

Figure 7.7 A Young Afran Qallo Woman with Kula made with Nail Polish

Applied polish, in contrast, promotes a more personal expression. Dabs of polish allow a young woman creative space to articulate an individual style that will catch the attention of a potential suitor she might meet on her way to and from market or on wood-gathering excursions. Decorating with polish also suggests high economic status. The price of an imported bottle of polish fetches the equivalent of four days' work for a wood or coal seller. Despite the cost, women are reluctant to collectively buy a bottle, since styles copied in a communal color from one face to another would not give the woman her unique look and promote her individual appeal.

As mentioned in Chapter One, polish is rarely wasted on the fingernails, since it is not an area that traditionally gets painted and, thus, not a candidate for the dissemination of cultural meaning. This again suggests women's astute decision to limit cosmetics to places on the skin that continue to be decorated in traditional ways. As a personal art, polish can literally exist alongside or on top of other kinds of markings that make resonant connections with collective Oromo values and belief systems.

Innovation and the Body Divided

Oromo women wear a range of necklaces, rings, bracelets, and hair ornaments made of colorful plastic and glass beads, shells, leather, amber, brass, tin, and silver filigree work. Women also apply temporary henna patterns and permanent tattoo designs to their hands, feet, faces, and gums; and dots of color to their cheeks and forehead with nail polish. When she can afford it, an Oromo woman has her upper incisors capped in gold and adds smudges of prepared kohl to her under-eye. Along with the medley of embroidered cotton, bright imported prints, and gauze scarves with which she covers her body and hair, an Oromo woman's costume embodies a rich accumulated, communicative aesthetic. First, ornament and dress reveal elements of her age, class, occupation, religious affiliation, and institutional membership. Secondly, her body adornment functions as a cultural map documenting historical, regional and lineage associations through style and form. Lastly, her attire provides avenues to define and adapt expressions of emergent ethnic identity.

Within this space, women as artists are governed by culturally endorsed prescriptions surrounding the degree to which innovation is encouraged or discouraged. In contrast, many Oromo body art consists of less permanent materials than other kinds of arts, such as carving and metalwork, and might therefore show more innovation. Further, among the Oromo and other patrilocal societies into which women move at marriage, new designs and techniques are transmitted with more frequency across regions than the arts of men. Yet, my research on dress suggests that there is considerable continuity in dress style throughout the historical periods under investigation. While young women who now have access to imported beads have experimented with innovative interlace headbands, their clothing styles, hair designs, and leather and metal jewelry have resisted drastic transformations in form and style. This push and pull in terms of innovation and dress, while at first perplexing, emerges out of a structured system based on Oromo notions of the body divided.

In some mask-carving traditions in West Africa, such as the Yoruba Gelede, the bottom face of a mask is always carved within a conventional style, while the superstructure is the place where the artist can freely play and innovate. In Oromo thought, the decoration of the female body is similarly constructed. It is at the upper torso where women are free to play, while the lower body resists new and innovative dress. *Kula* and *ambarka* are examples of the top transformation. The *saddetta* dress is only visible on the lower body where today its folds are reproduced in *maashiini*. A young woman will wear several innovative beaded necklaces, including *ambarka* decorated with safety pins and pieces of cardboard at her neck and on her chest (Figure 7.8). She also wears an imported T-shirt made in China in the color of her choice. Yet, around her waist she wears her *saddetta,* here fashioned as a skirt but identical to the lower dress worn four generations ago.

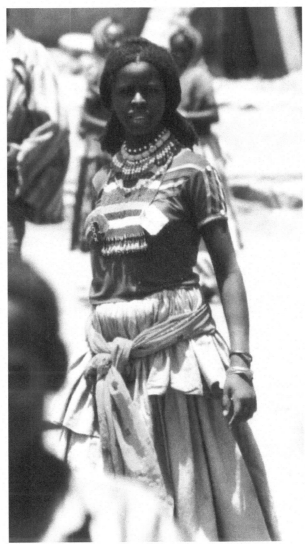

Figure 7.8 A Young Afran Qallo Woman wearing Ambarka, Imitation Amber, Paper Amulets, a Popular T-Shirt Imported from China, and Saddetta worn as a Skirt. She keeps the tuft of hair at the top of her head short until she is ready to marry

In her comparative piece on gendered dress among Kalabari and Americans, Eicher (2001, 246) finds that while the ideal body type in each case study is inherently different, in both the Nigerian and American cases, women are expected to display a sexed body through the exposure of skin. She writes that men's dress is named for their top garment while "the names for women's ensembles refer to the bottom items or garments that cover the genitalia, the reproductive site" (242). Like the Oromo, Kalabari women's dress is most closely associated with the lower body and its association with procreation. The lower body is connected to the past through its link to the ground, to birthing, and to concealment. The upper body is the seat of individuality where a layering of new forms is intended to catch the eye. Dress is a crucial component in the reconstruction of history, in the shaping of a nationalist ideology, and in the way that people make sense of themselves and their world. Herein, I have introduced body art practices that speak to the ways in which fashion in the form of constantly changing, imported commodities can be manipulated to reflect meaningful connections to indigenous notions of community, individuality, and memory. While the localized facial markings cut and dyed into the skin along the bridge of the nose, between the eyebrows and along the cheeks are being recast by bright pink and red nail polish, they are still embedded in the configuration of Oromo identity. Oromo women have developed a clear, cultivated fashion sense that connects them to people and places beyond their immediate communities but through the structure of Oromo dress codes. As one Oromo informant noted when asked how the Oromo maintain a sense of themselves through three generations of intense hardships, he remarked: "We teach our children to look for themselves in the subtle symbols carried by their mothers" (A.M., April 6, 2000).

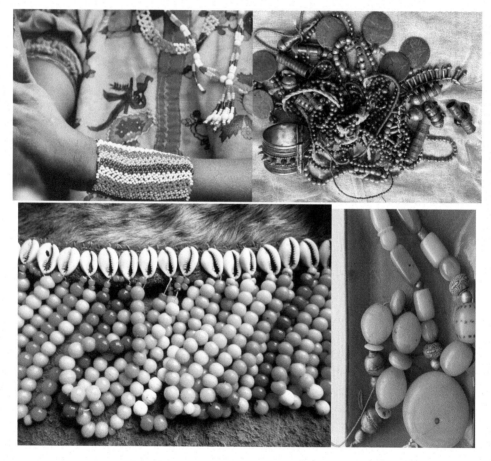

Figure 7.9 Oromo Beadwork and Metalwork

Endnotes

1   All translation errors are my own.

2   The Oromo Cultural Center does offer performances in the Oromo language for Oromo audiences, with actors clothed in the regional dresses of Oromia but events are first scripted to meet with administrative approval.

3   The Barentuma are divided into several subgroups who reside in the regions of Bale, Arsi, Hararghe, Shoa, and Wellega.

4   According to the Oromiya National Regions Government President Office, a population and housing census in 2007 recorded the population of Oromia at 27,158,471 and 36.7 percent of the population of Ethiopia. However, today this estimate is likely to be much higher.

5   As a foreign scholar writing about women and about art, I had a certain amount of autonomy once in the field in the early 2000s. It took four months in the capital to gain research clearance to conduct an Oromo project, and when I did travel beyond the confines of Harar for interviews and to film ceremonies, I was asked to have a member of the local Oromo cultural bureau present. Between 2003 and 2009, I was unable to secure research clearance.

6   A term first coined by the late African art historian Arnold Rubin (1974, 10).

7   Somali women in Jijjiga told me that it was in the 1980s that the majority of their silver, crescent-shape *audulli* necklaces were sold off to foreign collectors.

8   By focusing on a few dress types that hold significance as visible repositories of a tumultuous past, I resist writing an exhaustive listing of costume types that may either be unrelated to discussions of identity or that hold less historical merit. The data gathered on many different styles and forms of wear are a critical foundation for this and future writing, but since not all dress types carry the same value within Oromo society, many objects that may be momentarily fashionable are not considered in this study.

9   As recently as 1991, an Oromo council decided to use the Latin script rather than the dominant Amharic Sabean syllabary to write Afaan Oromo and, as of this writing, no unabridged English–Oromo dictionary of the language exists.

10 *Raba-dori* as a council should not be confused with *raba dori*, the fifth *gadaaa* grade.

11 While some discrepancy exists among scholars who have conducted genealogical studies among the Oromo, my data are most closely aligned with Kabir (1995) who conducted fieldwork on Afran Qallo history and genealogy. We differ substantially only in one major point. Where Kabir and Ibsa Ahmed places Qallo as the son of Hunbanna, I place Qallo as the adopted son of Barentuma once Akkichu is excommunicated (as illustrated in Figure 2.3). Gebissa and Kabir, respectively, record the four sons of Qallo as the Alla, Oborra, Baabile, and Daga *gossa*, and further divide the Daga into the Nole, Jarso, and Hume subclans or *warra* (Gebissa 2004, 34; Kabir 1995, 14). These divisions differ from earlier studies on the division of the Barentuma line (Ibsa Ahmed; Bahrey; Baxter; Braukämper; Haberland; Hassen; Waldron) but they stand in agreement with the division of the Qallo *gossa* with Brooke (1956) and my own findings. Kabir also found that the Barentuma branch of the great Oromo confederacy is referred to by the Afran

Qallo as 'Shanan Barentuma,' 'the Five Sons of Barentuma' (Kabir 1995, 8). While he remarks that 'Shanan Barentuma' is not cited by other scholars, I also found this term in use, particularly in reference to the *sabbata* discussed in Chapter Two (Kabir 1995, 7).

12   *Bishan jijjigo bahattin hin deebine*
      Akkichu Oromotti hin deebine

13   For a rich, comprehensive discussion of *moggaasaa*, see Hassen (2017, 156–158).

14   In fact, the wall surrounding Harar, thirteen to sixteen-and-a-half feet high and punctuated by five gates, is easily scaled and would not have kept a willing force from plundering the town. It is rather a visual symbol of the boundaries between the urban, Harari merchant society, and the predominantly Oromo farmers and agropastoralists outside the wall.

15   The reality of this account as an actual event of the tenth century is farfetched. Mohammed Hassen (1999, 4) has dismissed the presence of Oromo in Harar at the time of Shaykh Abadir in the tenth century as nothing more than a legend. To substantiate such a claim would require considerable archaeological and linguistic analysis that has not been carried out anywhere in the Central Highlands.

16   *Hunbannaa aayyaa Qunbii qabaayyaa*
      Murawwa aayaa Gawgaw irraa Ancaar qabaayyaa
      Xummuga aayaa Dida'aaf Baale qabaayyaa
      Karayyuu aayyaa Hadaamaaf Harsadee qabaayyaa
      Qallo aayyaa Cararii Balal qabaayyaa.

17   When I asked if Walaabuu referred to a specific place such as Haroo Walaabuu or Madda Walaabuu in Bale, informants only mentioned that it was an older place. It may be that, as Dereje Hinew (2012, 84) writes, Walaabuu references the original, landless water "out of which Waaqaa created all creatures." He writes:
      It was the place where human beings were continuously given all the necessary things from Waaqaa and people lived in peace. Walaabuu is perceived as a place of righteous and purity, a place where there was no unlawful activity, no suffering, and the place of truth and generally, the place where people were governed by the laws of Waaqaa. Therefore, the original Walaabuu seems to have been more related to cosmology than to a geographical area (85).

18   *Bariitee gargari gallaa.*

19   *Dagaa ayyaa wareeris qabaayyaa*
      Baabille ayyaa mullu qabaayyaa
      Obborra ayyaa Obbii qabaayyaa
      Allaa aabbaa mullata qabaayyaa.

20   Among the Arsi, Østebø (2009, 1054–1055) writes that women's belts are not only *wayyuu* (sanctified) but they "direct their prayers to the *ayyana hanfala laafa*" (the spirit of the soft belt). Women told her that the belt "expresses the spirit of all women as a collective marker."

21   This is further corroborated by Shell (2018).

22   *Chuchu* is probably a mishearing or miswriting by Paulitschke of '*huchu*' (clothing).

23   The neighboring Argobba are said to be the last group to give up the weaving of fine hairnets (*gufta*) that they wove on a small upright, wooden loom. One loom has been preserved in the Harari Cultural Museum but no Oromo looms exist in the region to my knowledge.

24   Along the coast, these bales were only fifteen thalers due to the shorter distance the cloth had to travel.

25   Burton also comments on the high quality of the Harari *tobe*s and sashes. This stands in opposition to the Egyptian officer Mohktar (quoted in Caulk 1977, 374) who writes that the Oromo wove a crude cloth and, therefore, sought out imported materials. The discrepancy in the description of the quality of locally woven cloth likely has much to do with Egyptian interest in creating a market for imported textiles.

26   Akou's description of the Somali *guntiino* dress made of seven cubits of cloth with a tie at the left shoulder and pleated may, in fact, be the *saddetta*. However, she writes: "A longer wrapped garment, called *saddexqayd*, was similar to the *guntinno* but used up to twenty yards of cloth." (Akou 2011, 35–36).

27   While the story of Tabo Mormo suggests that an outside group taught the Oromo to smelt, the Oromo probably also acquired the skill of using iron not from the Arabs, but from indigenous blacksmiths who were absorbed into the Oromo society through their *raba-dori* practice of adoption (M. Hassen, February 7, 2002).

28   *Faraasillaa bunaa manatti galchanii*
      Meetaa jaalataniis gamatti galchanii
      Kuula kuulaan hiitee kaantu-kaan caafamaa
      Kee manquuxiin hiitee kiyya na raafama. (S.A., April 4, 2000)

29   *Adareen ni gootii biyyon ni sossootii*
      Harkarra kilkillee laal addarra lootii
      Halaanaa Jijjigoo haroo Cinaaksanii
      Ardii lolaa kaate, numa qaqaysanii
      Dahab sifaa meeqaa meeta xalachanii.

30   An earlier draft of this chapter appears in *The Journal of Oromo Studies* 17(1) 2010: 111–135.

31   Men donning women's attire is not an unfamiliar phenomenon among other Cushitic pastoralists or groups organized around an age or generational grade system in East Africa. Among the Gabra Oromo in northern Kenya, too, male elders become classified as women and hold the responsibility for peace when they enter into a senior generational grade. They adopt women's dress styles and mannerisms (Wood 1999, 72). Among the Arsi Oromo, the Daballe and Gadaamojjii classes have been described as associated with the female character (see Østebø 2009, 1055).

32   Paulitschke (1888a, 50) estimates the Oromo populations he encountered to be as follows: 40,000 Nole, 60,000 Jarso, 100,000 Alla, 50,000 Ittu, and 20,000 Anniya.

33   The Ittu were one of the last groups in the regions to remain *wagafata* (*Waqaa*) practitioners (Ibsa Ahmed 2011, 23). Ittu women's leather dress may have served as a model for Afran Qallo women.

34   *Birraa birraa dararti baallii*
      sinnaara haarri akkami farri.

35   While the number of cattle here is based on the Nole *heera,* and is therefore approximate since it may change from one region to the next, the value ratio of the woman's breast is fixed among all Afran Qallo.

36   Prior to the rule by the Ethiopian state, *khat* was not a widespread crop among Afran Qallo Oromo farming communities (Gebissa 2004, 42–47). Harari tradition states that after the Battle of Calanzqoo where many Harari men perished, "their widowed wives, unable to tend to the khat, took the Kotus [Oromo] as tenants. The Kotus [Oromo] thus had the *khat* in their hands, and many gave the *khat* to their relatives to grow; thence the spread of *khat* on a widespread basis began." (Krikorian and Getahun 1973, 356). Oromo I spoke with maintain that they did chew *khat* before Calanqoo, but it was reserved for holy men and *wadaajaa* prayer ceremonies, where it could only be consumed by men and women over the age of forty years.

37   To be Amhara, as is the case among many ethnic groups, is therefore not a fixed ethnic category based on biological descent, but is a fluid cultural construct based largely on language, religion and cultural practice, including dress.

38   *Abban muka alaati, ayyoon utubaa manaati.*

39   Caulk (1971, 1) writes that Menelik's invasions of Oromo land in the late nineteenth century "parallel in their consequences the conditions created by contemporary acquisition of distant territories and peoples by the European powers." The intentional use of the terms 'conquest' and 'colonization' here to indicate the experiences of subjugation under Abyssinia as a colonial state, terms often reserved for European domination and forced rule over non-European nations has since the writing of Caulk become commonplace in scholarly writings on the Oromo. For further justification for the use of the term 'conquest' in this context and the common features of colonialism see Bulcha (1988, 35–61) and Holcomb and Ibssa (1990, 1–26).

40   See Kabir (1995) for a complete description of how laws were made and enforced in *heera gosa.*

41   Among the Arsi in eastern Bale, sexual crimes require eight cattle (M.T. Østebø 2009, 1056).

42 I was told that Maya Lama's name or that of her father can be found in the Arabic text *Fatul Habashat* where his reign is attributed to the seventeenth or eighteenth century, but I was not able to locate it there.

43 Gadid also mentions the legend of a Harari female ruler named 'Kamer', who was characterized as a warrior. Informants told him that she was the daughter of Aw Abdal, the Emir of Harar (1067–1086 B.C.E), though I could not corroborate this story of Kamer.

44 In Arsi communities, Waqaa practices are still observed and Kabir also mentions the interchange of Waqaa and Allah in Afran Qallo prayer. Among the Wallo in particular, it is considered the religion of the past. Today, *wadaajaa* is replaced with Mawlid or other Islamic celebrations. The occasion in which I heard the name 'Waqaa' used exclusively was during the Jiila ceremony in Jarso.

45 See Kumsa (1997) for an overarching discussion of the various roles *siiqee* plays in Oromo society.

46 Human Rights Watch reports that between mid-November 2016 and June 2016, Ethiopian security forces used excess and lethal force that resulted in 400 Oromo deaths and 10,000 being detained.

47 Like *ayyaana*, *atete* has many definitions. In Arsi, '*atete*' refers to an annual female water-centered ceremony that lasts one full day and night. The paraphernalia a woman uses is passed down from mother to daughter, and includes her stick, white clothing, jewelry, and food containers. The food and drink must be prepared without salt or sugar and the *marqa* must be made from only *garbuu* (barley) that has been soaked overnight and allowed to germinate. Prayers are offered by the participants that the coming year will be prosperous for people and their animals, and peace will prevail among family members. *Atete* is described by Trimingham (1965, 259) as an Oromo fertility goddess whose worship is survived by Muslims and Christians alike, while Morton (1973, 259–260) describes *atete* as a female divinity associated with the Virgin Mary and a female spirit known as 'Ayyaana Maryam.' Østebø (2009: 1053) mentions that *atete* and *siiqee* (*sinqee*) as interchangeable "refer both to religious marches as well as to political mobilizations conducted when women's rights or perhaps more correct to say, women's *wayyuu* has been violated." Also called '*delleqa*' in Hararghe, the *atete* ceremony in the past involved an exclusively female dancing and singing performance that today is publicly despised by Muslims who associate it as anti-Islamic.

48 Today, the Arabic term *karama* is more frequently used by the Oromo to describe this powerful energy of the wise and holy elderly transmitted as blessings through their saliva.

49 *Sadoon aayaa, sadoon ayyaa warar sadoo. Bishingaa gudee kan soolee, wararfaan boonaa kan Noole. Biyya dhirraa Gojoba.*

50 This reading of the social world of the living as replicated in the realm of spirits is also found in other African spirit sects such as the Hausa *bori* cult in northern Nigeria (see Masquelier).

51 Among the Borana, Bartels (1983, 287) surmises that the killing of the coffee bean is symbolic of the blood shed by women and connects to women and sexual intercourse. (For a detailed description of *buna qalla* among the Waso Borana, see Bassi (1998).)

52 Ibsa Ahmed (2011, 62) confirms that "the Itu regarded the Italian period as relief from oppression and exploitation."

53 *Lelee lelee, lelee, lelee*
    Suma danyaan biyya Roomaa jenerali
    Lelee lelee, lelee, lelee
    Shilingi tolchan Romaa.

54 There are ample examples in contemporary Africa, however, where hairstyle conveys other kinds of information. When the campaign slogan "Nigeria drive right" was implemented in 1972 to switch driving lanes, Yoruba women in southwest Nigeria were quick to create a hairstyle heavily weighted on the right, inspired by this slogan (Houlberg 1979, 349). In Central African urban centers, T. K. Biaya (1998, 85) reports that the modern fixation with wire-braiding came to replace "older concepts of beauty [while] rejecting forms of body decoration (such as tattooing, scarification and tooth-filing) which had served to mark the transition from childhood to puberty

and adulthood. The new regional fashion of wire-braiding later made way for wigs, whose success went hand in hand with 'xessal' or 'ambi' (skin-lightening)."

55   This is not true among other ethnic groups. In Gambela in southwestern Ethiopia, it is only after marriage and a child that women have their heads shaved, thus signaling their maturity and their ability to participate more fully in social and political affairs. Before their children come, Anuwak and Nuer women in Gambela wear sculptural, asymmetrical hairstyles that mirror the patterns of the clay pipes that they smoke for recreation. The shaving of the head may also be connected to mourning in the Ethiopian Northern Highlands.

56   One of the most influential studies of hair in non-Western societies, written in the late 1950s by Leach (1958), suggests that to manipulate the hair is subconsciously sexual. Based on the psychoanalytical readings of Berg, Leach's (1958) theory states that head hair is symbolically equivalent to pubic hair and that the cutting of the hair thus corresponds to castration. Ten years later, this theory is challenged by Hallpike (1969, 258) who cites, for example, the frequency with which women shave or cut their head hair. Instead, he proposes that "long hair is associated with being outside society [as in the case of priests] and that the cutting of hair symbolizes re-entering society, or living under a particular disciplinary regime within society" (260). The fact that Oromo women used to have their head shaved at their infibulation ceremony, which deals directly with the cutting of their sex and the restriction of their sex drive, suggests, at first glance, that Leach's model may well be appropriate as an analytical method. However, Oromo women that I spoke with do not articulate any symbolic connections between their haircutting, either at infancy or at puberty, with sex or castration. Instead, their shaved heads are intended to communicate their liminal healing period and virginity

57   Interestingly, Finneran (2011, 62) mentions that to protect against those with the evil eye, the Arsi Oromo construct "counter-charms from large frames of wood and the pudenda of ritually slaughtered cattle and place them at crossroads." Further evidence of the significant power bestowed upon the human and animal vagina might be found in Oromo pastoralist communities.

58   The notion that only females who are "properly" women, that is, those who have begun menstruating and have undergone either excision or initiation can marry is upheld in several African societies. The association with this state of being reproductively sound and the tying of cloth at the waist, resonates in Northeast Africa and in West Africa. For instance, among Kalabari women in Rivers State, Nigeria, the lifecycle that begins with menses was referred to as bite *pakiri iwain* (tying half the length of a piece of cloth), while *konju fina* (waist tying stage) demonstrated that a Kalabari female was old enough to tie cloth at the waist, and had attained maturation of her reproductive capabilities" (Michelman and Erekosima 1992, 174, 175).

59   *Faraasillaa bunaa manatti galchanii*
      Meetaa jaalataniis gamatti galchanii
      Kuula kuulaan hiitee kaantu-kaan caafamaa
      Kee manquuxiin hiitee kiyya na raafama. (S.A., April 4, 2000).

60   Another version of the origin of the *gufta* that circulates among the Harari is that this hairstyle was created in the fifteenth century by a Portuguese queen. The legend states that she came with the Portuguese army, married a Harari emir, and converted to Islam. Since she wanted to maintain her Christian heritage, at least at a symbolic level, she made three demands of the Harari people. First, she asked that a cross be incorporated into the house architecture. Second, she told the tailors to include an embroidered cross pattern at the bottom of Harari women's gowns. Third, she asked that women's hair be worn in two balls on either side of their neck so that in silhouette their head, hair, and neck would become the shape of a cross (Ahmed Zekaria, October 12, 1999).

61   Concrete linguistic evidence would certainly help to determine from where the *gufta* originated. While Gibb (1996, 343) attributes the word '*gufta*' to the Oromo language, the Oromo linguist that I spoke with did not think it came originally from Afaan Oromo. Further, the term '*hamasha*' used to describe the hairstyle is unlikely to have come from any spoken Ethiopian language. It was suggested to me that '*hamasha*' is of East Indian origin, but I have been unable to locate it, as yet, in modern Indian languages. It may be an indigenous Oromo term (M. Hassen, February

22, 2002).

62   My translation from the German.

63   This wood is called '*lullutii*' in the Argobba language.

64   Orthodox Christian women in Ethiopia also cover their hair and torso in public with a hand-woven, gauze-like cloth called a '*shamma*.' Oromo women say that their cloth and style of wear is in accordance with Islamic tradition, and is different from their Amhara neighbors.

65   Oromo women wear their two balls of hair toward the back, behind the shoulder and Harari women keep their *gufta* directed forward. Harari women also tend to wear the more expensive kinds of *gufta*, namely those finely woven and hand-embroidered with colorful yarn or metallic threads. While both Oromo and Harari women wear *gufta*, the quality of materials and their styles of wear create two distinct kinds of hairdressings.

66   *Ya isi ilmon qabne.*
      Ak' sin teese tschoptu! (My translation from the German.)

67   Since many practicing Muslim Oromo assert that Islam frowns upon the exchange of the bride for material goods, the bride price has decreased in the last decade. The only sanctioned gifts, as stated in the Qur'an, are the animals and/or money from the groom to the bride (*maharii*). In marked contrast to the traditional Oromo wedding, Shari'a law also forbids dancing, and requires the separation of men and women during the ceremony.

68   For a description of the eight types of marriages recognized and practiced among the Arsi Oromo, see Jemila Adem.

69   *Intalaa haadhuun deemtu miti, Intala haadaan deemtu, Rabbi han godhu.*

70   *Ilmaniin sii deema, Ilmaafii sitti deema na seensisii.*

71   *Si offolchee seenii, arkadhu gabbadhu.*

72   *Fuudha intalaa siiqqee milkii, fuudha qurbaa bordoo milkii.* This saying is still repeated during the engagement ceremony today in Baabile when the elders untie the bundles of *khat* leaves as a symbol of agreement.

73   *Daboo aayaa baabaloo aayyaa siin dibaa laali. Akkuma raaseen dibe mataa kee, maal gadi baasuun dhibdhe abbaa kee, Akkuma raaseen dibe martii tee laal gad si baasuun dhibde lammi tee. Abbittoon kankee geegayoo foohatee ayyiyyoo taantee garaan foolatee.*

74   *Mudattee heera, sabbatan jabeeysi garaa.* The fiancé is responsible for providing this *sabbata* and the cloth to wear over her *saddetta*. He must also provide her female friends with *marinka*, a sash worn over the left shoulder over the *saddetta* and tied around the waist. This sash is worn by the bride's maids when they go the to the bride's house on the first day of the marriage ceremony.

75   The practice of keeping sharp metal objects near a newborn can be found throughout North Africa. Becker (2011, 62) reports that an Amazigh child in Morocco is given a necklace with a silver knife pendant.

76   Oromo national consciousness is largely informed by a debate centered on whether the Oromo in their nation of Oromia should attempt to secede from the Ethiopian state or rally for equal treatment and self-determination as members of a unified Ethiopia. This contemporary debate surrounding self-determination and/or secession has largely been organized and theorized outside of Ethiopia in the Oromo Diaspora and published in the likes of I.M. Lewis (ed) *Nationalism and Self-Determination in the Horn of Africa* 1983, Baxter, Hultin and Triulzi (eds), *Being and Becoming Oromo* (1996), and Jalata, *Oromo Nationalism and the Ethiopian Discourse* (1998).

77   The Orthodox Christian origin myth has been used by the Amhara and Tigrean Semitic groups to legitimate their control of the country. They link themselves to the Solomonic dynasty in Jerusalem from which Haile Selassie, the last emperor of Ethiopia, is said to have been the final biological descendant. Legend narrates that the Queen of Sheba (Sabea) visited Solomon, the King of Jerusalem and son of King David, and from their encounter bore a son, Menelik I. As a young man, Menelik I returned to Jerusalem and was crowned Emperor of Ethiopia by his father. On his return to Ethiopia, he stole the Ark of the Covenant and placed it in the Church at Axum, St. Mary of Zion. With the covenant and the blood of Solomon in the house, the way was cleared for Menelik I and his biological heirs to rule by divine right. Menelik II (1889–1913) was named after this legendary leader. The Amhara since the time of Axum, have tripled their

empire through imperialistic endeavors, and encouraged a national identity by 'Amharacizing' other ethnic groups through the spread of the Amharic language, custom and religion.

78   See, for example, Bonnie Holcomb and Sisai Ibssa, *The Invention of Ethiopia: The Making of a Dependent Colonial State in Northeast Africa 1990 and Contested Terrain; The Invention of Ethiopia*. Ezekiel Gebissa, (ed.), *Contested Terrain. Essays on Oromo Studies, Ethiopianist Discourse, and Politically Engaged Scholarship*, 2009.

79   Paulitschke (1896, 162) also finds it strange that the Somali, the Afar and the Oromo seem never to have tried to reproduce human images, animal figures, or vegetal forms in jewelry or on household objects.

80   The braided hairstyle of an unmarried girl. This line refers to the movement of the *naannoo*. If the head movement is abrupt, it makes the sound '*fash.*' If the head is gently rotated, the sound of the *naannoo* is referred to as wave-like and designated as '*lash*' or '*raph*' (Guutamma Ammallee, March 1, 2002).

81   The singer is particularly admiring the area between the eyes that is often scarred, tattooed or decorated with dabs of nail polish.

82   The two meanings for *kula* apply here. *Kula* (to apply color) can refer to the blue-black pigment used as eyeliner and as a tattooing substance or it may signify the threads or fibers worn around a woman's forehead (Taman Youssoff, February 26, 2002).

83   The beaded headband of a young Oromo woman.

84   Metal crescent-shaped earrings.

85   A necklace made of circular shaped metal beads.

86   Two younger women I interviewed who lived in Harar did express shame at their facial tattoos, stating that it was forbidden by Allah (I.M. and D.A., March 28, 2000). It may be that facial tattooing begins to wane in the future. The practice among Moroccan Amazigh women as reported by Becker (2006b, 48) has disappeared due to Islamic influence.

Bibliography

Abbink, Jon. *Ethiopian Society and History: A Bibliography of Ethiopian Studies, 1957–1990*. Leiden: African Studies Centre, 1990.

———. "Ch'at in Popular Culture: A 'Prayer' from Harār, Ethiopia." *Sociology Ethnology Bulletin* 1 No. 2 (1992): 89–93.

Abdallah, Imran. "A History of Harar Town (1900 to the Early 1930s)." BA thesis, Addis Ababa University, 1997.

Abdurahman, Abdulla. "Harari Funeral Customs Part 1." *Ethnological Society Bulletin* 1 No. 2 (1953): 1–4.

———. "Harari Funeral Customs Part 2." *Ethnological Society Bulletin* 1 No. 1 (1953): 23–26.

———. "Harari Wedding Customs Part 1." *Ethnological Society Bulletin* 1 No. 2 (1953): 4–8.

———. "Harari Wedding Customs Part 2." *Ethnological Society Bulletin* 1 No. 3 (1954): 22–26.

Abir, Mordechai. "Brokerage and Brokers in Ethiopia in the First Half of the 19th Century." *Journal of Ethiopian Studies* 3 No. 1 (1965): 1–5.

———. "The Contentious Horn of Africa." *Conflict Studies*, vol. 24. London: Institute for the Study of Conflict, 1972.

———. *Ethiopia and the Red Sea: The Rise and Decline of the Solomonic Dynasty and Muslim–European Rivalry in the Region*. London u.a.; Cass, 1980.

Adem, Jemila. "Women and Indigenous Conflict Resolution Institutions in Oromia: Experience from *Siinqee* of the Wayyu Shanan Arsi Oromo in Adami Tulla Jiddu Kombolcha District of the Ormia National Regional State." Master's thesis, Addis Ababa University, 2014.

Aguilar, Mario I. "Waaso Boorana Women's Theology: A Silent Journey." *Feminist Theology* 5 (1994): 40–57.

———. *Being Oromo in Kenya*. Trenton: Africa World Press, 1998.

Ahmed, Abbas. "A Historical Study of the City–State of Harar (1795–1875)." Master's thesis, Addis Ababa University, 1992.

Ahmed, Ibsa. *The Eastern Oromo in the 19th and 20th Centuries.* Germany: Lap Lambert Academic Publishing, 2011.

Ahmed, Yusuf Ali. "An Inquiry Into the Household Economy of the Amirs of Harar 1925–1875." *Ethnological Society Bulletin* 1 No. 10 (1960): 7–62.

Akou, Heather. *The Politics of Dress in Somali Culture.* Bloomington: Indiana University Press, 2011.

Allman, Jean, ed. *Fashioning Africa: Power and the Politics of Dress.* Bloomington; Indianapolis: Indiana University Press, 2004.

Appadurai, Arjun, ed. *The Social Life of Things.* Cambridge: Cambridge University Press, 1986.

Aquilar, M. I. "Recreating a Religious Past in a Muslim Setting: 'Sacrificing' Coffee–Beans Among the Waso Boorana of Garba Tull, Kenya." *Ethnos* 60 nos 1–2 (1995): 41–58.

Ardener, Shirley. *Women and Space: Ground Rules and Social Maps.* New York: St. Martin's Press, 1981.

Arnoldi, Mary Jo, and Christine Mullen Kreamer. *Crowning Achievements: African Arts of Dressing the Head.* Los Angeles: Fowler Museum of Cultural History University of California Los Angeles, 1995.

Aronson, Lisa. "Threads of Thought: African Cloth as Language." In *African and African-American Sensibility*, edited by Michael W. Coy, Jr. and Leonard Plotnicov, 67–90. Pittsburgh: University of Pittsburgh, 1995.

Arthur, Linda B. *Religion, Dress and the Body.* Oxford: Berg, 1999.

Azais, R. P. and Chambard, R. *Cinq Annees de Recherches Archeologiques en Ethiopie: Province de Harar Et Ethiopie Meridionale.* Paris: Librarie Orientaliste: Paul Geuthner, 1931.

Bachem, Bele. "Weissgekleidetes Harar." *Merian* 19 (1966): 60–67.

Bahrey, Abba, and Manoel de Almeida, G.W.B. Huntingford, and C.F. Beckingham. *History of the Galla (Oromo) of Ethiopia: With Ethnology and History of South-West Ethiopia.* Oakland: African Sun, 1993.

Baissa, Lemmu. "Contending Nationalisms in the Ethiopian Empire State and the Oromo Struggle for Self–Determination." In *Oromo Nationalism and the Ethiopian Discourse*, edited by Asafa Jalata, 79–108. Lawrenceville: The Red Sea Press, 1998.

Bamberger, Joan. "The Myth of Matriarchy: Why Men Rule in Primitive Society." In *Woman, Culture, and Society*, edited by Michelle Zimbalist Rosaldo, Louise Lamphere, and Joan Bamberger, 263–80. Stanford: Stanford University Press, 1974.

Bann, Stephen. *The Clothing of Clio: A Study of the Representation of History in Nineteenth-Century Britain and France.* New York: Cambridge University Press, 1984.

Bardey, Alfred. "Notes Sur Le Harar." *Imprimerie Nationale* (1900): 130–180.

Barker, W. C. "Extract. Report on the Probable Geographical Position of Harrar; with Some Information Relative to the Various Tribes in the Vicinity." *Journal of the Royal Geographical Society of London* 12 (1842): 238–244.

Barnes, Ruth, and Joanne Bubolz Eicher. *Dress and Gender: Making and Meaning in Cultural Contexts.* New York: Berg: St. Martin's Press, 1992.

Barnes, Virginia Lee, and Janice Patricia Boddy. *Aman: The Story of a Somali Girl.* 1st American ed. New York: Pantheon Books, 1994.

Bartels, Lambert. "Dabo: A Form of Cooperation Between Farmers Among the Macha Galla." *Anthropos* 70 (1975): 883–889.

———. *Oromo Religion: Myths and Rites of the Western Oromo of Ethiopia: An Attempt to Understand.* Collectanea Instituti Anthropos, vol. 8. Berlin: D. Reimer, 1983.

Basha, Ejetta Feyessa. "Newcomers and the People of Harar in the Early 20th Century." Paper prepared for the Conference on Harari Studies organized by the Historical Society of Ethiopia. Addis Ababa, 1975. 1–8.

Bassi, Marco. *I Borana: Una Società Assembleare Dell'etiopia.* Antropologia Culturale E Sociale, vol. 42. Milano: F. Angeli, 1996.

———. "Every Woman an Artist. The Milk Containers of Elemu Boru." In *Ethiopia. Traditions of Creativity*, edited by Raymond Silverman, 65–87. Seattle: University of Washington Press, 1999.

Baxter, P. T. W. "Atete in a Highland Arssi Neighborhood." *Northeast African Studies* 1 (1979): 1–22.

———. "The Problem of the Oromo or the Problem for the Oromo." In *Nationalism and Self-Determination in the Horn of Africa*, edited by I. M. Lewis, 129–150. Ithaca; London: Ithaca Press, 1983.

———. "Some Observations on the Short Hymns Sung in Praise of Shaikh Nur Hussein of Bale." In *The Diversity of the Muslim Community: Anthropological Essays in Memory of Peter Lienhardt*, edited by Ahmed Al-Shahi, 139–152. London: Published for the British Society for Middle Eastern Studies by Ithaca Press, 1987.

Baxter, P. T. W., and Uri Almagor. *Age, Generation, and Time: Some Features of East African Age Organisations.* New York: St. Martin's Press, 1978.

Baxter, P. T. W. Jan Hutlin and Alessandro Triulzi. *Being and Becoming Oromo: Historical and Anthropological Enquires.* Lawrence; Asmara: The Red Sea Press, 1996.

Becker, Anne E. *Body, Self, and Society: The View from Fiji*. Philadelphia: University of Pennsylvania Press, 2013.

Becker, Cynthia. *Amazigh Arts in Morocco, Women Shaping Berber Identity*. Austin: University of Texas Press, 2006a.

———. "Amazigh Textiles and Dress in Morocco." *African Arts* 39 No. 3 (2006b): 42–96.

Beckwith, Carol, and Angela Fisher. *African Ceremonies*. New York: Harry N. Abrams, 1999.

Beckwith, Carol, Angela Fisher, and Graham Hancock. *African Ark: Peoples of the Horn*. London: Collins Harvill, 1990.

Behrend, Heike, and Ute Luig. *Spirit Possession, Modernity and Power in Africa*. Madison: University of Wisconsin Press, 1999.

Beidelman, T. O. *The Cool Knife: Imagery of Gender, Sexuality, and Moral Education in Kaguru Initiation Ritual*. Washington: Smithsonian Institution Press, 1997.

Beke, Charles T. "Observations on the Road from Tajurah to Schoa." *Journal of the Royal Geographical Society of London* 12 (1842): 238–244.

Berhanesellasie, Tsehai. "Menelik II. Conquest and Consolidation of the Southern Provinces." B.A. thesis. Addis Ababa University, 1969.

Biasio, Elisabeth, Zehirun Yetmgeta, Girmay Hiwet, Worku Goshu, Peter R. Gerber, and Wolfgang Bender. *Die Verborgene Wirklichkeit: Drei Äthiopische Maler Der Gegenwart, Zerihun Yetmgeta, Girmay Hiwet, Worku Goshu*. Zürich: Völkerkundemuseum der Universität Zürich, 1989.

Biaya, T. K. "Hair Statements in Urban Africa: The Beauty, the Mystic and the Madman." *The Art of African Fashion*. 75–101. Asmara: African World Press, 1998.

Blackhurst, Hector. "Continuity and Change in the Shoa Galla Gada System." In *Age Generation and Time*, edited by P. T. W. Baxter, and Uri Almagor, 151–82. London: C. Hurst, 1978.

Boddy, Janice Patricia. *Wombs and Alien Spirits: Women, Men, and the Zar Cult in Northern Sudan*. Madison, Wis.: University of Wisconsin Press, 1989.

Braukämper, Ulrich. "Oromo Country of Origin: A Reconsideration of Hypothesis." *Proceeding of the Sixth International Conference of Ethiopian Studies* (1980): 25–40.

———. "Notes on the Islamization and the Muslim Shrines of the Harar Plateau." *Proceedings of the Second International Congress of Somali Studies*. Hamburg: Buske Verlag, 145–74. vol. 2, 1983.

Bricchett-Robecchi, L. *Nell'harar*. Milano: Casa Editor, 1896.

Bridgwood, Ann. "Dancing the Jar: Girls' Dress at Turkish Cypriot Weddings." In *Dress and Ethnicity: Change Across Space and Time,* edited by Ruth and Joanne Eicher Barnes, 29–51. Washington: Oxford Press, 1995.

Brøgger, Jan. *Belief and Experience Among the Sidamo: A Case Study Towards an Anthropology of Knowledge.* Oslo; Oxford: Norwegian University Press; Oxford University Press, 1986.

Brooke, Clarke Harding. "Settlements of the Eastern Galla, Hararghe Province, Ethiopia." Ph.D. dissertation. University of Nebraska, 1956.

Buckridge, Steeve O. *The Language of Dress: Resistance and Accommodation in Jamaica, 1760–1890.* Jamaica: University of the West Indies Press, 2004.

Bulcha, Mekuria. *Flight and Integration: Causes of Mass Exodus from Ethiopia and Problems of Integration in the Sudan.* Uppsala: Scandinavian Institute of African Studies, 1988.

———. "The Survival and Reconstruction of Oromo National Identity." In *Being and Becoming Oromo*, edited by P. T. W. Baxter, Jan Hutlin, and Alessandro Triulzi, 48–66. Lawrenceville; Asmara: The Red Sea Press, 1996.

Burton, Richard F. "Narrative of a Trip to Harar." *Journal of the Royal Geographical Society of London* 25 (1855): 136–50.

———. *First Footsteps in East Africa, or, an Exploration of Harar,* edited by Isabel Burton, New York: Dover, 1987.

Buschkens, Willem F. L., and L. J. Slikkerveer. *Health Care in East Africa: Illness Behaviour of the Eastern Oromo in Hararghe (Ethiopia).* Assen, The Netherlands: V. Gorcum, 1982.

Buxton, David Roden. *Travels in Ethiopia.* New York: F. A. Praeger, 1967.

Capotti, M. "Usi E Constumi Galla." *L'Esploratore* (1883): 101–03.

Cassanelli, Lee V. "Qat: Changes in the Production and Consumption of a Quasi–Legal Commodity in Northeast Africa." In *The Social Life of Things: Commodities in Cultural Perspective*, edited by A. Appadurai, 236–57. Cambridge: Cambridge University Press, 1986.

Caulk, Richard. "The Occupation of Harar: January 1887." *The Journal of Ethiopian Studies* 9 No. 2 (1971): 1–19.

———. "Menilek's Conquest and Local Leaders in Harar." Paper prepared for the Conference on Harari Studies organized by the Historical Society of Ethiopia, Addis Ababa, 1975. 1–15.

———. "Harar Town in the Nineteenth Century and Its Neighbours in the Nineteenth Century." *Journal of African History* 18 No. 3 (1977): 369–86.

Cavallaro, Dani, and Alexandra Warwick. *Fashioning the Frame: Boundaries, Dress, and Body.* New York: Berg, 1998.

Cerulli, Enrico. "Documenti Arabi per La Storia dell' Ethiopia." *Memorie della Reale Academia dei Lincei* 4. Roma: G. Bardi (1931): 37-101.

———. *La Lingua E La Storia Di Harar Studi Etiopici*. Pubblicazioni Dell'istituto Per L'oriente. Roma: Istituto per l'Oriente, 1936.

Chojnacki, Stanislaw. "Notes on Art in Ethiopia in the 15th and 16th Century" *Journal of Ethiopian Studies* 8 (1970): 21–65.

———. "Two Ethiopian Icons" *African Art* 12 (1977): 44–51, 87.

Cole, Herbert M., and University of California Santa Barbara. Art Gallery. *African Arts of Transformation*. Santa Barbara: University of California, 1970.

Coleman, James Smoot, and Richard L. Sklar. *Nationalism and Development in Africa: Selected Essays*. Berkeley: University of California Press, 1994.

Condee, Nancy. "Body Graphics: Tattooing the Fall of Communism." In *Consuming Russia*, edited by Adele Marie Barker, 339–61. Durham: Duke University Press, 1999.

Connerton, Paul. *How Societies Remember*. Themes in the Social Sciences. Cambridge [United Kingdom]; New York: Cambridge University Press, 1989.

Conrad, David C., and Barbara E. Frank. *Status and Identity in West Africa Nyamakalaw of Mande*. Bloomington: Indiana University Press, 1995.

Cotter, George. *Proverbs and Sayings of the Oromo People of Ethiopia and Kenya with English Translations*. African Studies, vol. 25. Lewiston, N.Y.: E. Mellen Press, 1992.

———. *Ethiopian Wisdom: Proverbs and Sayings of the Oromo People*. African Proverbs Series, vol 1. Ibadan; Daystar: Sefer, 1996.

Crapanzano, Vincent, and Vivian Garrison. *Case Studies in Spirit Possession*. New York: Wiley, 1977.

Dahl, Gudrun. "Possession as Cure: The Ayaana Cult among the Waso Borana." In *Culture, Experience and Pluralism*, edited by Anita Jacobson-Widding, and D. Westerlund, 151–65. Vol. 14. Uppsala: Uppsala Studies in Cultural Anthropology, 1989.

Das Is Abessinien, L'abyssinie Telle Qu'elle Est. Bern; Leipzig; Wien: Wilhelm Goldmann Berlag, 1935.

de Salviac, Martial. *Un Peuple Antique au Pays de Menelik: Les Galla Grande Nation Africain*. Paris: H. Oudin, 1905.

Debsu, Dejene N. "Gender and Culture in Southern Ethiopia: An Ethnographic Analysis of Guji–Oromo Women's Customary Rights." *African Study Monographs* 30 No. 1 (2009): 15–36.

Deressa, Belletech. *Oromtitti: The Forgotten Women in Ethiopian History*. Raleigh: Ivy House, 2003.

Deressa, Daniel. "Continuity and Changes in the Status of Women: The Case of Arsi Oromo Living Adjacent to Upper Wabe Valley (Dodola)." Master's thesis, Addis Ababa University, 2002

Donham, Donald L. *Work and Power in Maale, Ethiopia*. 2nd ed. New York: Columbia University Press, 1994.

————. *Marxist Modern: An Ethnographic History of the Ethiopian Revolution*. Berkeley; Oxford: University of California Press; J. Currey, 1999.

Donham, Donald L., and W. James, eds., *The Southern Marches of Imperial Ethiopia: Essays in History and Social Anthropology*. Cambridge: Cambridge University Press, 2002.

Drewal, Henry John, and Margaret Thompson Drewal. *Gelede: Art and Female Power Among the Yoruba*. Bloomington: Indiana University Press, 1993.

Drewal, Margaret Thompson. *Yoruba Ritual: Performers, Play, Agency*. Bloomington: Indiana University Press, 1992.

Eicher, Joanne B. "Dress, Gender and the Public Display of Skin." In *Body Dressing*, edited by Joanne Entwistle and Elizabeth Wilson, 233–252. Oxford: Berg, 2001.

Eicher, Joanne B., and Mary Ellen Roach–Higgins. "Definition and Classification of Dress: Implications for Analysis of Gender Roles." In *Dress and Gender: Making and Meaning in Cultural Contexts*, edited by R. Barnes and J. Eicher, 8–28. Rhode Island: Berg, 1992.

Entwistle, Joanne. *The Fashioned Body: Fashion, Dress, and Modern Social Theory*. Cambridge: Malden: Polity Press, 2000.

————. "The Dressed Body." In *Body Dressing*, edited by Joanne Entwistle, and Elizabeth Wilson, 33–58. Oxford: Berg, 2001.

Eshete, Almeme. "The Establishment of the Capuchin Catholic Mission Among the Qottu of Harar. 1881–1889." Paper presented at the Conference on Harari Studies organized by the Historical Society of Ethiopia, Addis Ababa, 1975. 1–13.

Farago, Ladislas. *Abyssinia on the Eve*. New York: G.P. Putnam's Sons, 1935.

Fernandez, James W. "Principles of Opposition and Vitality in Fang Aesthetics." *Journal of Aesthetics and Art Criticism* 25 (1966): 53–64.

Finneran, Niall. "Ethiopian Evil Eye Belief and the Magical Symbolism of Iron Working." *Folklore* 114 No. 3 (2003): 427–433.

Fischer, Eberhardt, and Hans Himmelheber. *The Arts of the Dan of West Africa*. Switzerland: AG Bern, 1976.

Fisher, Angela. *Africa Adorned*. New York: Abrams, 1984.

Freeman, Dena, and Alula Pankhurst, eds. *Peripheral People: The Excluded Minorities of Ethiopia*. London: Hurst, 2003.

Forbes, Rosita Torr. *From Red Sea to Blue Nile: Abyssinian Adventure*. New York: The Macaulay Company, 1925.

Foucher, E. "Une Inscription Hindi au Sanctuaire de Sheikh Abadir (Harar)." *Quaderni di Studi Etiopici* 5 (1984): 96–99.

———. "The Cult of Muslim Saints in Harar: Religious Dimension." In *Proceedings of the 11th International Conference of Ethiopian Studies*, edited by R. Pankhurst and T. Beyene Bahru Zewde, 71–83. Addis Ababa, 1994.

Fritzsche, G. "Die Karawanenstrasse von Zeila Nach Ankober." *Geographische Mittheilungen* Heft 5 (1890): 113–18.

Fukui, Katsuyoshi, and John Markakis. *Ethnicity and Conflict in the Horn of Africa*. London: James Currey, 1994.

Gadid, Mahdi. "Feudalism in the Emirate of Harar up to 1887." Senior thesis, Addis Ababa University, 1979.

Galaty, John G., and Pierre Bonte. *Herders, Warriors, and Traders: Pastoralism in Africa*. African Modernization and Development Series. Boulder: Westview Press, 1991.

Gamta, Tilahun. *Oromo–English Dictionary*. Addis Ababa: AAU Printing Press, 1989.

Garad, Abd al-Rahman. *Wirtschaft Geschichte Eines Emirates im Horn von Afrika, 1825–75*. Frankfurt: Lang, 1990.

Gebissa, Ezekiel. *Leaf of Allah: Khat and Agricultural Transformation in Harerge Ethiopia, 1875–1991*. Oxford: James Currey, 2004.

———, ed., *Contested Terrain: Essays on Oromo studies, Ethiopianist Discourse, and Politically Engaged Scholarship*. Trenton; Asmara: Red Sea Press, 2009.

Gebrechristos, Berhane. "The Municipality of Harar: An Appraisal of Its Inhabitations and Prospects." BA thesis, Addis Ababa University, 1972.

Gell, Alfred. *Wrapping in Images: Tattooing in Polynesia*. Oxford: New York: Clarendon Press; Oxford University Press, 1993.

Gerster, George. *Churches in Rock: Early Christian Art in Ethiopia*. London: Phaidon Press, 1970.

Gibb, Camilla. "Religion, Politics and Gender in Harar, Ethiopia." PhD dissertation, University of Oxford, 1996.

———. "Constructing Past and Present in Harar." In *Ethiopia in Broader Perspective: Papers of the 13th International Conference of Ethiopian Studies*, edited by Eisei Kurimoto, Katsuyoshi Fukui, and Masayoshi Shigeta, 378–90. Kyoto, 1997.

———. "Sharing the Faith: Religion and Ethnicity in the City of Harar." *Horn of Africa* 16 nos. 1–4 (1998): 144–62.

———. "Baraka without Borders: Integrating Communities in the City of Saints." *Journal of Religion in Africa* 29 No. 1 (1999): 88–108.

Giles, Linda. "Spirit Possession and the Symbolic Construction of Swahili Society." In *Spirit Possession. Modernity and Power in Africa*, edited by Heike Behrend, and Ute Luig, 142–164. Madison: The University of Madison Press, 1999.

Gleichen, Count Edward. *With the Mission to Menelik, 1897*. London: Edward Arnold, 1898.

Gnamo, Abbas Haji, "Islam, the Orthodox Church and Oromo Nationalism (Ethiopia)." *Cahiers d'études Africaines* 165 (2002): 99–120.

Gnisci, Jacopo. "An Ethiopian Miniature of the Tempietto in the Metropolitan Museum of Art: Its Relatives and Symbolism." In *Canones: The Art of Harmony; The Canon Tables of the Four Gospel*, edited by A. Bausi, B. Reudenbach, and H. Wimmer, 67–98. Berlin; Boston: De Gruyter, 2020.

———. "Christian Metalwork in Early Solomonic Ethiopia: Production, Function, and Symbolism." In *Peace, Power, and Prestige: Metal Arts in Africa*, edited by S. Cooksey, 254–265. Gainesville, Florida: University Press of Florida, 2020.

Gott, Suzanne. "Asante Hightimers and the Fashionable Display of Women's Wealth in Contemporary Ghana." *Fashion Theory: The Journal of Dress, Body & Culture* 13 No. 2 (2009): 141–176.

Gragg, Gene B., and Kumsa Terfa. *Oromo Dictionary*. [Ethiopian Series]. Monograph Committee on Northeast African Studies, No. 12. East Lansing: African Studies Center Michigan State University in Cooperation with Oriental Institute University of Chicago, 1982.

Greenfield Richard and Hassen, Mohammed. "The Oromo Nation and Its Resistance to Amhara Colonial Administration." In *Proceedings of The First International Congress of Somali Studies*, edited by Hussein M. Adam and Charles I. Geshekter, 546–599. Atlanta: Scholars Press, 1992.

Hallpike, C.R. "Social Hair." *Man* 4 No. 2 (1969): 256–64.

Hamer, John and Irene. "Spirit Possession and Its Socio-Psychological Implications Among the Sidamo of Southwest Ethiopia." *Ethnology* 5 (1966): 392–408.

Haberland, Eike. *Galla Süd-*Äthiopiens. Stuttgart: Kohlhammer, 1963.

Harbeson, John W. *The Ethiopian Transformation: The Quest for the Post–Imperial State*. Boulder: Westview Press, 1988.

Hardin, Kris L. *The Aesthetics of Action: Continuity and Change in a West African Town*. Washington: Smithsonian Institution Press, 1993.

Harris, Corn Wallis. *The Highlands of Ethiopia*. London: Longman, 1844.

Hassan, Salah M. "Henna Mania: Body Painting as a Fashion Statement, from Tradition to Madonna." In *The Art of African Fashion,* 103–131. Asmara: African World Press, 1998.

Hassen, Mohammed. "The Relation Between Harar and the Surrounding Oromo Between 1800–1887." BA thesis, Haile Selassie University, 1973.

———. "Menelik's Conquest of Harar, 1887, and Its Effect on the Political Organization of the Surrounding Oromos up to 1900." *Working Papers on Society and History in Imperial Ethiopia: The Southern Periphery from the 1880s to 1974,* edited by D. L. Donham, and Wendy James, 227–246. Cambridge: African Studies Center: 1980.

———. "The Oromo of Ethiopia, 1500–1850: With Special Emphasis on the Gibe Region." PhD dissertation, University of London, 1983.

———. *The Oromo of Ethiopia: A History, 1570–1860.* Cambridge; New York: Cambridge University Press, 1990.

———. "The Development of Oromo Nationalism." In *Being and Becoming Oromo,* edited by P. T. W. Baxter, Jan Hutlin, and Alessandro Triulzi, 67–80. Lawrenceville; Asmara: The Red Sea Press, 1996.

———. "The Machu–Tulama Association and the Development of Oromo Nationalism." In *Oromo Nationalism and the Ethiopian Discourse,* edited by Asafa Jalata, 183–221. Asmara: The Red Sea Press, 1998.

———. "The City of Harar and the Islamization of the Oromo in Hararghe, 1550s–1900." Paper presented at the African Studies Association Meeting. Philadelphia, 1999.

———. "Islam as Resistance Ideology among the Oromo of Ethiopia." In *Africa, Islam and Development: Islam and Development in Africa,* edited by Thomas Saeter, and Kenneth King, 79–114. Edinburgh: Centre of African Studies, University of Edinburgh, 2000.

———. Personal Communication. February 22, 2002.

———. "Pilgrimage to the Abbaa Muudaa." *The Journal of Oromo Studies* 12 nos. 1/2 (2005): 142–155.

———. "The Egyptian Occupation of Harer and Its Impact on the Oromo of Harerge." *The Journal of Oromo Studies* 15 No. 2 (2008): 33–66.

———. *The Oromo and the Christian Kingdom of Ethiopia 1300–1700.* Woodbridge: James Currey, 2017.

Hassen, Mustefa. "Culture on Transition: A Case of Adare (Harari) Ethnic Group." BA thesis, Addis Ababa University, 1988.

Healy, Sally. "The Changing Idiom of Self-Determination in the Horn of Africa." In *Nationalism and Self-Determination in the Horn of Africa,* edited by I. M. Lewis, 93–109. London: Ithaca Press, 1983.

Hecht, Elisabeth–Dorothea. "The Voluntary Associates and the Social Status of Harari Women." *Sixth International Conference of Ethiopian Studies*, 295–308. Tel Aviv, 1980.

————. "The City of Harar and the Traditional Harari House." *Journal of Ethiopian Studies* 15 (1982): 56–78.

————. "Basketwork of Harar." *African Studies Monographs* (October 1992): 1–39.

Heldman, Mariyln. *African Zion: The Sacred Arts of Ethiopia*. New Haven: Yale University Press, 1996.

Hendrickson, Hildi. *Clothing and Difference: Embodied Identities in Colonial and Post-Colonial Africa*. Durham; London: Duke University Press, 1996.

Henige, David P. *The Chronology of Oral Tradition; Quest for a Chimera*. Oxford Studies in African Affairs. Oxford: Clarendon Press, 1974.

Henze, Paul B. *Ethiopian Journeys: Travels in Ethiopia 1969–1972*. London: Tonbridge Ernest Benn, 1977.

Hicks, Esther K. *Infibulation: Female Mutilation in Islamic Northeastern Africa*. New Brunswick: Transaction Publishers, 1993.

Hinew, Dereje. "Historical Significances of Odaa with Special Reference to Walaabuu." *Star Journal*, April–June 1 No. 2 (April–June 2012): 81–90.

Hinnant, John. "Spirit Possession, Ritual and Social Change: Current Research in Southern Ethiopia." *Rural Africana* (1970): 107–111.

————. "The Guji: Gada as a Ritual System." In *Age Generation and Time: Some Features of East African Age Organisations*, edited by P. T. W. Baxter and Uri Almagor, 207–243. London: C. Hurst, 1978.

————. "The Position of Women in Guji Oromo Society." In *Proceedings of the 8th International Conference of Ethiopian Studies*, edited by Taddese Beyene, 799–808. Addis Ababa, 1984.

————. "Ritualization of the Life Cycle." In *New Methods for Old Age Research*, edited by Christine Fry, and Jennie Keith, 163–184. Massachusetts: J. F. Bergin Publishers, 1986.

————. "Ritual and Inequality in Guji Dual Organization." In *The Attraction of Opposites: Thought and Society in a Dualistic Mode*, edited by David May-Bury Lewis, and Uri Almagor, 57–76. Ann Arbor: University of Michigan Press, 1989.

————. "Guji Trance and Social Change: Symbolic Responses to Domination." *Northeast African Studies* 12 No. 1 (1990): 65–78.

Hobsbawm, E. J. *Nations and Nationalism Since 1780: Programme, Myth, Reality*. Cambridge; New York: Cambridge University Press, 1990.

Holcomb, Bonnie, and Peri Klemm. "The Matter of Land is a Matter of Life. *'Dubbiin Lafaa, Dubbii Lafeeti'*: Examining Cultural Messaging in an Oromo Protest Song, 'Ka'i Qeerroo.'" *The Journal of Oromo Studies* 25 (2018): 63–97.

Holcomb, Bonnie K., and Sisai Ibssa. *The Invention of Ethiopia: The Making of a Dependent Colonial State in Northeast Africa*. Trenton: Red Sea Press, 1990.

Hollander, Anne. *Seeing Through Clothes*. New York: Avon, 1980.

Houlberg, Marilyn Hammersley. "Social Hair: Tradition and Change in Yoruba Hairstyles in Southwestern Nigeria." In *The Fabrics of Culture*, edited by Justine M. Cordwell, and Ronald A. Schwarz, 349–397. The Hague: Mouton Publishers, 1979.

Huntingford, G. W. B. *The Glorious Victories of 'Amda Ṣeyon, King of Ethiopia*. Oxford: Clarendon Press, 1965.

———. *The Galla of Ethiopia: The Kingdoms of Kafa and Janjero*. London: International African Institute, 1969.

Jalata, Asafa. *Oromia and Ethiopia: State Formation and Ethnonational Conflict, 1868–1992*. Boulder: L. Rienner, 1993.

———. "The Emergence of Oromo Nationalism and the Ethiopian Reaction." In *Oromo Nationalism and the Ethiopian Discourse: The Search for Freedom and Democracy*, edited by Asafa Jalata, 1–26. Lawrenceville; Asmara: Red Sea Press, 1998.

———. *Contending Nationalisms of Oromia and Ethiopia: Struggling for Statehood, Sovereignty, and Multinational Democracy*. Binghamton: Global Academic Publishing, 2010.

Kabir, Bedri. "The Afran Qallo Oromo. A History." BA thesis, Addis Ababa University, 1995.

Karp, Ivan. "Power and Capacity in Iteso Rituals of Possession." In *Personhood and Agency: The Experience of Self and Other in African Cultures*, edited by Michael Jackson, and Ivan Karp, 79–94, vol. 14. Uppsala; Washington: Uppsala University; Distributed by Smithsonian Institution Press, 1990.

Kasfir, Sidney L. Kasfir. *African Art and the Colonial Encounter: Inventing a Global Commodity*. Bloomington: Indiana University Press, 2007.

Kassam, Aneesa, and Gemetchu Megersa. "Iron and Beads: Male and Female Symbols of Creation: A Study of Ornament among Booran Oromo." In *The Meaning of Things: Material Culture and Symbolical Expression*, edited by I. Hodder, 23–31. London: Allen and Unwim, 1989.

Kassam, Aneesa, and Ali Balla Bashuna. "Marginalisation of the Waata Oromo Hunter Gatherers of Kenya: Insider and Outsider Perspectives" *Africa* 74 No. 2 (2004): 194–216.

Keller, Edmond. "Regime Change and Ethno-Regionalism in Ethiopia: The Case of the Oromo." In *Oromo Nationalism and the Ethiopian Discourse*, edited by Asafa Jalata, 79–108. Lawrenceville: The Red Sea Press, 1998.

Kinfu, Johannes. "The Anteregnoch in Ethiopia: Jewelers from Axum; Role and Status in a Peasant Society and Transitional Economy." In *Ethiopia in Broader Perspective: Papers of the 13th International Conference of Ethiopian Studies*, edited by Eisei Kurimoto, Katsuyoshi Fukui, and Masayoshi Shigeta, 71–77. Kyoto, 1997.

Kirk, R. "Reports on the Route from Tajurra to Ankobar, Travelled by the Mission to Shoa, Under the Charge of Captain W. Harris, 1841." *Journal of the Royal Society of London* 12 (1842): 221–238.

Klemm, Peri M. "Two Corporeal Markers of Marriage among the Afran Qallo Oromo Women in Eastern Ethiopia." *Proceedings of the 15th International Conference of Ethiopian Studies*, edited by S. Uhlig, 136–141. Addis Ababa, Ethiopia, 2006.

———. "Leather Amulets in Ethiopia" In *Faith and Transformation: Votive Offerings and Amulets from the Alexander Girard Collection*, edited by Doris Francis, 98–100. Girard Collection, Museum of International Folk Art, Museum of New Mexico Press, 2007.

———. "Oromo Fashion: Three Contemporary Body Art Practices Among Afran Qallo Women." *African Arts* 42 No. 1 (2009): 54–63.

———. "Tying Oromo History: The Manipulation of Dress during the Late Nineteenth Century." *The Journal of Oromo Studies* 17 No. 1 (2010): 111–135.

———. "We Grew Up Free but Here We Have to Cover Our Faces." Veiling Among Oromo Refugees in Eastleigh, Kenya. In *Veiling in Africa*, edited by Elisha Renne, 186–204. Bloomigton: Indiana University Press, 2013.

———. "Unrest and Dress: The Symbol of the Sycamore Tree in Oromo Adornment." In *Creating African Fashion Histories: Politics, Museums and Sartorial Practice*, edited by JoAnn McGregor, Heather Akou, Nicola Stylianou, and Lou Taylor. Indiana University Press, Forthcoming.

Klemm, Peri M. and Barbie Campbell Cole. 2003. "Historical Threads: An Overview of Women's Dresses in Harar." *Archiv fur Volkerkunde* 53 (2003): 63–72.

Klemm, Peri M., and Leah Niederstadt. "Beyond Wide-Eyed Angels: Contemporary Expressive Culture in Ethiopia." *African Arts* 42 No. 1 (2009): 6–13.

Klumpp, Donna, and Corinne Kratz. "Aesthetics, Expertise and Ethnicity: Okiek and Maasai Perspectives on Personal Ornament." In *Being Maasai: Ethnicity and Identity in East Africa*, edited by Thomas Spear, and Richard Waller, 195–221. London: James Curry Ltd., 1993.

Klopper, S. "Re-Dressing the Past: The Africanization of Sartorial Style in Contemporary South Africa." In *Hybridity and Its Discontents: Politics, Science, Culture*, edited by A. Brah and A. E. Coombes, 216–232. London: Routledge, 2000.

Knutsson, K. E. *Authority and Change: A Study of the Kallu Institution Among the Macha Galla of Ethiopia*. Goteborg: Elanders Boktryskari Aktiebolag, 1967.

Kramer, Fritz. *The Red Fez: Art and Spirit Possession in Africa*. London; New York: Verso, 1993.

Kratz, Corinne Ann. *Affecting Performance: Meaning, Movement, and Experience in Okiek Women's Initiation*. Washington: Smithsonian Institution Press, 1994.

Kratz, Corinne, and Donna Pido. "Gender, Ethnicity and Social Aesthetics in Maasai and Okiek Beadwork." In *Rethinking Pastoralism in Africa: Gender, Culture and the Myth of the Patriarchal Pastoralist*, edited by Dorothy L. Hodgson, 43–71. Oxford: James Currey, 2000.

Krikorian, Amare Getahun and A. D. "*Chat*: Coffee's Rival Form Harar, Ethiopia; Botany, Cultivation and Use." *Economic Botany* 27 (1973): 353–377.

Kumsa, Martha Kuwee. "The *Siiqqee* Institution of Oromo Women." *The Journal of Oromo Studies* 4 (1997): 115–152.

————. "Oromo Women and the Oromo National Movement: Dilemmas, Problems and Prospects for True Liberation." In *Oromo Nationalism and the Ethiopian Discourse*, edited by Asafa Jalata, 153–182. Lawrenceville; Asmara: Red Sea Press, 1998.

————. *Songs of Exile. Singing the Past Into the Future*. Kitchener: Duudhaa Publishing, 2013.

————. "Precarious Positioning: Tensions in Doing *Siiqqee* Feminist Social Work Research." In *Feminisms in Social Work Research* edited by Stephanie Wahab, Ben Anderson-Nate, and Christina Gingeri, 154–169. Oxford: Routledge, 2014.

Lambek, Michael Joshua. *Knowledge and Practice in Mayotte: Local Discourses of Islam, Sorcery and Spirit Possession*. Toronto: University of Toronto Press, 1993.

Last, Jill, "Hairstyles Today." *Selamta* 12 No. 2 (1995): 14–18.

Last, Jill and Nancy Donovan. *Ethiopian Costumes*. Addis Ababa, Ethiopia: Ethiopian Tourism Commission, 1980.

Laurence, Margaret. *New Wind in a Dry Land*. 1st American ed. New York: Knopf, 1964.

Leach, Edmund. "Magical Hair." *Journal of the Royal Anthropological Insitute* 88 No. 2 (1958): 147–64.

Legesse, Asmarom. *Gada: Three Approaches to the Study of African Society.* New York: Free Press, 1973.

Leiris, Michel. "La Croyance Aux Genies 'Zar' En Ethiopie du Nord." *Jornal de Psychologie* 1–2, (1938): 108–126.

Levine, Donald Nathan. *Greater Ethiopia: The Evolution of a Multiethnic Society.* Chicago: University of Chicago Press, 1974.

Lewis, Herbert S. *A Galla Monarchy; Jimma Abba Jifar, Ethiopia, 1830–1932.* Madison: University of Wisconsin Press, 1965.

———. "The Origin of the Galla and Somali." *Journal of African History* 6 No. 1 (1966): 27–46.

———. "Spirit Possession in Ethiopia: An Essay in Interpretation." In *Proceedings of the 7th International Conference of Ethiopian Studies*, edited by S. Rubenson, 419–427. Lund, Sweden, 1982.

Lewis, I. M. "The Galla of Northern Somaliland." *Rassegna di Studi Etiopici* 15 (1959): 21–38.

———. Introduction to *Nationalism and Self Determination in the Horn of Africa.* London: Ithaca Press, 1983.

———. *A Modern History of Somalia: Nation and State in the Horn of Africa.* Westview Special Studies in Africa, rev., updated, and expanded ed. Boulder: Westview Press, 1988.

———. *Ecstatic Religion: A Study of Shamanism and Spirit Possession.* 2nd ed. London; New York: Routledge, 1989.

———. *Saints and Somalis: Popular Islam in a Clan-based Society.* Lawrenceville, NJ: Red Sea Press, 1998.

Lewis, I. M., Ahmed El Safi, and Sayed Hamid A. Hurreiz. *Women's Medicine: The Zar–Bori Cult in Africa and Beyond.* Edinburgh: Edinburgh University Press for the International African Institute, 1991.

Lindisfarne, Nancy, and Bruce Ingham. *Languages of Dress in the Middle East.* Richmond, Surrey: Curzon in Association with the Centre of Near and Middle Eastern Studies SOAS, 1997.

Loughran, Katheryne S. *Somalia in Word and Image.* Washington, D.C.: Published by the Foundation for Cross-Cultural Understanding in Cooperation with Indiana University Press Bloomington, 1986.

Loughran, Kristyne, and Edith Suzanne Gott. *Contemporary African Fashion.* Bloomington: Indiana University Press, 2010. eBook Academic Collection (EBSCOhost). Web. 4 July 2016.

Marcus, Harold G. *A History of Ethiopia.* Berkeley: University of California Press, 1994.

Markakis, John. *National and Class Conflict in the Horn of Africa*. Cambridge: New York: Cambridge University Press, 1987.

Masquelier, Adeline. "Mediating Threads: Clothing and the Texture of Spirit/ Medium Relations in Bori (Southern Niger)." In *Clothing and Difference: Embodied Identities in Colonial and Postcolonial Africa*, edited by Hildi Hendrickson, 66–93. Durham; London: Duke University Press, 1996.

———. "The Invention of Anti–Tradition." In *Spirit Possession: Modernity and Power in Africa*, edited by H. Behrend, and U. Luig, 34–49. Madison: The University of Madison Press, 1999.

———. *Prayer Has Spoiled Everything: Possession, Power, and Identity in an Islamic Town of Niger*. Durham: London: Duke University Press, 2001.

Massaja, Guglielmo. *I Miei Trentacinque Anni Di Missione Nell'alta Etiopia; Memorie Storiche di Fra Guglielmo Massaja*, vol. 3. Milan: Tipografia S. Giuseppe, 1886.

McKay, Roger. "Ethiopian Jewelry." *African Arts* 7 No. 2 (1974): 36–39.

Megerssa, Gemetchu. "Oromumma: Tradition, Consciousness and Identity." In *Being and Becoming Oromo: Historical and Anthropological Enquiries*, edited by Jan Hutlin, Alessandro Triulzi, and P. T. W. Baxter, 92–102. Lawrenceville; Asmara: The Red Sea Press, 1996.

———. "The Oromo and the Ethiopian State Ideology in a Historical Perspective." In *Papers of the 13th International Conference of Ethiopian Studies*, edited by Eisei Kurimoto, Katsuyoshi Fukui, and Masayoshi Shigeta, 479–485. Kyoto, 1997.

Melbaa, Gadaa. *Oromia: An Introduction*. 2nd ed: privately printed, 1988.

Mercier, Jacques. *Art That Heals: The Image as Medicine in Ethiopia*. Munich; New York, N.Y.: Prestel; Museum for African Art, 1997.

———. *Ethiopian Magic Scrolls*. New York: George Braziller, 1979.

Messing, Simon. D. "Group Therapy and Social Status in the Zar Cult of Ethiopia." *American Anthropologist* 60 (1958): 1120–1125.

———. "The Non-Verbal Language of the Ethiopian Toga." *Anthropos* 55 nos. 3/4 (1960): 558–560.

Michelman, Susan O., and Tonye V. Erekosima. "Kalabari Dress in Nigeria: Visual Analysis and Gender Implications." In *Dress and Gender: Making and Meaning*, edited by Ruth Barnes, and Joanne B. Eicher, 164–182. Providence; Oxford: Berg, 1992.

Mohktar, Muhammad. "Notes sur le Pays de Harrar." *Bulletin de la Societe Khediviale de Geographie* 5 (1876): 351–97.

Moore, Eine. *Jewelry*. Ethiopian Tourist Commission. Addis Ababa: Commercial Press, 1975.

Morton, Alice. "Some Aspects of Spirit Possession in Ethiopia." PhD dissertation, University of London, 1973.

Muudee, Mahdi Hamid. *Oromo Dictionary*. Atlanta, Georgia: Sagalee Oromoo Publishing Co. Inc., 1995.

Natvig, Richard. "Oromos, Slaves, and the Zar Spirits: A Contribution to the History of the Zar Cult." *The International Journal of African Historical Studies* 20 No. 4 (1987): 669–689.

Nicholl, Charles. *Somebody Else: Arthur Rimbaud in Africa, 1880–91*. Chicago: The University of Chicago Press, 1997.

Ornter, Sherry. "Is Female to Male as Nature to Culture?" In *Woman, Culture, and Society*, edited by Joan Bamberger, Louise Lamphere, and Michelle Zimbalist Rosaldo, 67–87. Stanford: Stanford University Press, 1974.

Østebø, Marit Tolo. "Wayyuu Women's Respect and Rights Among the Arsi Oromo." In *Proceedings of the 16th International Conference of Ethiopian Studies*, edited by S. Ege, H. Aspen, B. Teferra, and S. Bekele, 1049–1060. Trondheim: NTNU-trykk, 2009.

Owens, Jonathan. *A Grammar of Harar Oromo (Northeastern Ethiopia)*. Hamburg: H. Buske, 1985.

Pankhurst, Richard. "Harar at the Turn of the Century." *Ethiopia Observer, Special Issue on Harar* 2 No. 2 (1958): 62–65.

———. *An Introduction to the Economic History of Ethiopia, from Early Times to 1800*. London: Lalibela House, 1961.

———. "The Harar–Dire Dawa Road and the 'Road Construction Association' of 1934." Addis Ababa: Paper submitted to the Historical Society of Ethiopia Conference, 1975.

———. *History of Ethiopian Towns from the Mid-Nineteenth Century to 1935*. F. Steiner Verlag Wiesbaden, 1985.

———. *A Social History of Ethiopia: The Northern and Central Highlands from Early Medieval Times to the Rise of Emperor Téwodros II*. 1st American ed. Trenton: Red Sea Press, 1992.

———. *The Ethiopian Borderlands: Essays in Regional History from Ancient Times to the End of the 18th Century*. Lawrenceville: Red Sea Press, 1997.

Pankhurst, Silvia. "Harar under Egyptian Rule" *Ethiopia Observer: Special Issue on Harar* 2 No. 2 (1958a): 56–58.

———. "A Visit to Harar." *Ethiopia Observer: Special Issue on Harar* 2 No. 2 (1958b): 34–43.

Paulitschke, Philipp. "Le Harar Sous L'administration Egyptienne, 1875–1885." *Bulletin Societe Khedive Geographie* 10 No. 2 (1887): 575–91.

———. *Beiträge Ethnographie Und Anthropologie der Somâl, Galla und Harari.* Leipzig: Verlag von Eduard Baldmus, 1888a.

———. *Harar; Forschungsreise Nach den Somal Und Gallaländern, Ost-Afrikas.* Leipzig: F. A. Brockhaus, 1888b.

———. "Die Wanderung Der Oromo." *Geographische Mitteilungen der Anthropologischen Gesellschaft* (1889): 166–178.

———. *Ethnographie Nordost–Afrikas: Die Geistige Cultur der Danakil, Galla Und Somal.* Berlin: Geographische Verlagschandlung Dietrich Reimer, 1896.

Pennebaker, James W., Darío Páez, and Bernard Rimé. *Collective Memory of Political Events: Social Psychological Perspectives.* Mahwah, N.J.: Lawrence Erlbaum Associates, 1997.

Perani, Judith, and Fred T. Smith. *The Visual Arts of Africa: Gender, Power, and Life Cycle Rituals.* Upper Saddle River: Prentice Hall, 1998.

Perani, Judith, and Norma Hackleman Wolff. *Cloth, Dress, and Art Patronage in Africa.* Oxford; New York: Berg, 1999.

Perczel, C. F. "Ethiopian Painting: Sources, Causes and Effects of Foreign Influences in the Sixteenth and Seventeenth Centuries" *Proceedings of the Seventh International Conference of Ethiopian Studies*, University of Lund: 1984, 165–175.

Plowden, Walter Chichele. *Travels in Abyssinia and the Galla Country with an Account of a Mission to Ras Ali in 1848.* London: Longmans, Green, and Co., 1868.

Rasmussen, Susan J. "Spirit Possession and Personhood Among the Kel Ewey Tuareg." *Cambridge Studies in Social and Cultural Anthropology.* Vol. 94. Cambridge; New York: Cambridge University Press, 1995.

———. *Healing in Community: Medicine, Contested Terrains, and Cultural Encounters Among the Tuareg.* Westport, Conn.: Bergin & Garvey, 2001.

Ravenhill, Philip L. *The Art of the Personal Object: Exploring African Art.* 1st Harper–Perennial ed. Seattle, Washington: National Museum of African Art, 1991.

Reclus, Elisee. *Nouvelle Geographie Universelle; la Terre et les Hommes.* Paris: Libraire hachette et cie, 1885.

Reminick, Ronald A. "The Evil Eye Belief Among the Amhara of Ethiopia." *Ethnology* 13 (1974): 279–291.

Renne, Elisha P. *Cloth That Does Not Die: The Meaning of Cloth in Bùnú Social Life.* Seattle: University of Washington Press, 1995.

Riesman, Paul. "The Person and the Life Cycle in African Social Life and Thought." *African Studies Review* 29 (1986): 71–138.

Rikitu, Mengesha. *Oromia Recollected*. London: Magic Press, 1998.

Rimbaud, Jean-Nicolas-Arthur. "To the Bosphore Égyptien." (1887). Translated by Mark Spitzer. In *Exquisite Corpse: A Journal of Letters and Life* 5/6 (1999). http://www.corpse.org/issue_5/secret_agents/rimbaud.htm

Roach, Mary Ellen, and Joanne Bubolz Eicher. *Dress, Adornment, and the Social Order*. New York: Wiley, 1965.

———. "The Language of Personal Adornment." In *The Fabrics of Culture: The Anthropology of Clothing and Adornment*, edited by Justine M. Cordwell, and Ronald A. Schwarz, 7–21. The Hague; Paris; New York: Mouton, 1979.

Roach–Higgins, Mary Ellen, Joanne Bubolz Eicher, and Kim Karen Johnson. *Dress and Identity*. New York: Fairchild Publications, 1995.

Robecchi-Bricchetti, L. *Nell'Harar*. Milano: Casa Editr. Galli, 1896.

Robinson, Cedric J. "The African Diaspora and the Italo–Ethiopian Crisis." *Race & Class* 17 No. 2 (October 1985): 51-65.

Rosaldo, Michelle Zimbalist. "Woman, Culture, Society: A Theoretical Overview." In *Woman, Culture, and Society*, edited by Michelle Zimbalist Rosaldo, Louise Lamphere, and Joan Bamberger, 17–42. Stanford: Stanford University Press, 1974.

Ross, Heather Colyer. *The Art of Bedouin Jewellery: A Saudi Arabian Profile*. 3rd ed. Montreux, Switzerland: Arabesque, 1989.

Rovine, Victoria L. *Bogolan: Shaping Culture Through Cloth in Contemporary Mali*. Bloomington: Indiana University Press, 2008

Rubin, Arnold. *African Accumulative Sculpture: Power and Display*. New York: Pace Gallery, 1974.

Rugh, Andrea B. "Reveal and Conceal: Dress in Contemporary Egypt." *Contemporary Issues in the Middle East*. 1st ed. Syracuse: Syracuse University Press, 1986.

Salt, Henry. *A Voyage to Abyssinia in the Years 1809 and 1810*. London: Longmans, 1844.

Samatar, Said S. *Oral Poetry and Somali Nationalism*. Cambridge: University of Cambridge Press, 1982.

Schlee, Günther. *Oromo Nationalist Poetry*. Working Paper/Universität Bielefeld, Fakultät Für Soziologie, Forschungsschwerpunkt Entwicklungssoziologie, No. 174. Bielefeld, Germany: Universität Bielefeld, 1992.

Schneider, Jane, and Annette B. Weiner. *Cloth and Human Experience*. Washington: Smithsonian Institution Press, 1989.

Sciama, Lidia D., and Joanne Bubolz Eicher. *Beads and Bead Makers: Gender, Material Culture, and Meaning*. Oxford; New York: Berg, 1998.

Shack, William A. "Hunger, Anxiety, and Ritual: Deprivation and Spirit Possession in among the Gurage of Ethiopia." *Man* 6 (1971): 30–43.

Sharp, Lesley Alexandra. *The Possessed and the Dispossessed: Spirits, Identity, and Power in a Madagascar Migrant Town*. Berkeley: University of California Press, 1993.

Shell, Sandra Rowoldt. *Children of Hope: The Odyssey of Oromo Slaves from Ethiopia to South Africa*. Ohio University Press, 2018.

Shiferaw, Berhane. "The Marriage Custom of the Adare Society Since the Italian Invasion." BA thesis, Addis Ababa University, 1982.

Sieber, Roy. "Prelude." In *Hair in African Art and Culture* edited by Roy Sieber, Frank Herreman, and Niangi Batulukisi, 15–17. New York; Munich: Museum for African Art; Prestel, 2000.

Sieber, Roy, Roslyn A. Walker, and National Museum of African Art (U.S.). *African Art in the Cycle of Life*. Washington, D.C.: Published for the National Museum of African Art by the Smithsonian Press, 1987.

Silverman, Raymond A., ed., *Ethiopia: Traditions of Creativity*. Lansing: Michigan State University Museum; Seattle: University of Washington Press, 1999.

Silverman, Raymond A., and Neal Sobania. "Icons of Devotion/Icons of Trade: Creativity and Entrepreneurship in Contemporary 'Traditional' Ethiopian Painting," *African Arts* 42 No. 1 (2009): 26–37.

Simak, Evelyn, and Carl Dreibelbis. *African Beads: Jewels of a Continent*. Denver: Africa Direct, 2010.

Slikkerveer L J. *Plural Medical Systems in the Horn of Africa: The Legacy of Sheik Hippocrates*. London; New York: Kegan Paul International, 1990.

Sorenson, John. *Imagining Ethiopia: Struggles for History and Identity in the Horn of Africa*. New Brunswick: Rutgers University Press, 1993.

Spencer, Paul. *Nomads in Alliance; Symbiosis and Growth Among the Rendille and Samburu of Kenya*. London; New York: Oxford University Press [for the School of Oriental and African Studies], 1973.

Starkie, Enid. *Arthur Rimbaud in Abyssinia*. Oxford Studies in Modern Languages and Literature. Oxford: The Clarendon Press, 1937.

Stenning, Derrick J. *Savannah Nomads: A Study of the Wodaabe Pastoral Fulani of Western Bornu Province, Northern Region, Nigeria*. London: Published for the International African Institute by Oxford University Press, 1959.

Stroomer, Harry. *A Grammar of Boraana Oromo (Kenya): Phonology, Morphology, Vocabularies*. Köln: R. Köppe, 1995.

Sumberg, Barbara. "Dress and Ethnic Differentiation in the Niger Delta." In *Dress and Ethnicity: Change across Space and Time*, edited by J. Eicher, 165–182. Washington: Oxford Press, 1995.

Sumner, Claude. *Oromo Wisdom Literature*. Addis Ababa: Gudina Tumsa Foundation, 1995.

———. *Proverbs, Songs, Folktales: An Anthology of Oromo Literature*. Addis Ababa: Gudina Tumsa Foundation, 1996.

Synnott, Anthony. *The Body Social: Symbolism, Self and Society*. London; New York: Routledge, 1993.

Swayne, H. G. C. *Seventeen Trips Through Somaliland and a Visit to Abyssinia: A Record of Exploration and Big Game Shooting, with Descriptive Notes on the Fauna of the Country*. 3rd ed. London: Rowland Ward, 1895.

Talle, Aud. "Transforming Women into 'Pure' Agnates: Aspects of Female Infibulation in Somalia." In *Carved Flesh/Cast Selves. Gendered Symbols and Social Practices*, edited by Vigdis Broch-Due, Ingrid Rudie, and Tone Bleie, 83–106. Oxford: Berg, 1993.

Tamene, Bitima, and Jürgen Stueber. *Die Ungelöste Nationale Frage in Äthiopien: Studie zu den Befreiungsbewegungen der Oromo und Eritreas*. Frankfurt am Main: P. Lang, 1983.

Taye, Eshete. "Marriage and Family Among the Deder Oromo, Harrarghie Region." BA thesis, Addis Ababa University, 1984.

Tesfaye, Andargachew. "The Funerary Customs of the Kottu of Harar." *Ethnological Society Bulletin* 7, (1957): 35–40.

Thesiger, Wilfred. *The Danakil Diary: Journeys Through Abyssinia, 1930–34*. London: HarperCollins, 1996.

Thompson, Robert Farris. *African Art in Motion*. Los Angeles; Berkeley; London: University of California Press, 1974.

Tonkin, Elizabeth. *Narrating Our Pasts: The Social Construction of Oral History*. Cambridge; New York: Cambridge University Press, 1992.

Torrey, E. Fuller. "The Zar Cult in Ethiopia." *International Journal of Social Psychiatry* 13 No. 3 (1967): 216–223.

Trimingham, J. Spencer. *Islam in Ethiopia*. London: Frank Cass, 1965.

Triulzi, Alessandro. "Competing Views of National Identity in Ethiopia." In *Nationalism and Self-Determination in the Horn of Africa*, edited by I. M. Lewis, 111–127. London: Ithaca Press, 1983.

Turner, Bryan S. *The Body and Society: Explorations in Social Theory*. Oxford: Basil Blackwell, 1985.

Turner, Victor Witter, and Richard Schechner. *The Anthropology of Performance*. New York: PAJ Publications, 1986.

Vale, Lawrence J. *Architecture, Power, and National Identity*. New Haven: Yale University Press, 1992.

Valentia, George Viscount. *Voyages and Travels to India, Ceylon, the Red Sea, Abyssinia, and Egypt*. London: Bulmer and Co., 1809.

van de Loo, Joseph. *Guji Oromo Culture in Southern Ethiopia: Religious Capabilities in Rituals and Songs*. Berlin: Dietrich Reimer Verlag, 1991.

van Gennep, Arnold. *The Rites of Passage*. Chicago: University of Chicago Press, 1960.

Vansina, Jan. *Oral Tradition as History*. Madison: University of Wisconsin Press, 1985.

———. "Afterthoughts on the Historiography of Oral Tradition." In *African Historiographies: What History for Which Africa?*, edited by Bogumil Jewsiewicki, and David S. Newbury, 105–110, Beverly Hills: Sage Publications, 1986.

Vivian, Herbert. *Abyssinia. Through the Lion-Land to the Court of the Lion of Judah*. London: Arthur Pearson Ltd., 1901.

Wagner, Ewald. "Three Arabic Documents on the History of Harar." *Journal of Ethiopian Studies* 12 No. 1 (1974): 213–224.

Waldron, Sidney R. "Social Organization and Social Control in the Walled City of Harar, Ethiopia." PhD dissertation, Columbia University, 1974.

———. "The Political Economy of Harari–Oromo Relationships, 1559–1874." *Northeast African Studies* 6 nos. 1/2 (1984): 23–39.

———. "Within the Wall and Beyond: Harari Ethnic Identity and Its Future." In *Urban Life: Readings in Urban Anthropology*, edited by G. Gmelch, and W. Zenner, 249–256. New York: St. Martin's Press, 1980.

Wellby, Nontagu Sinclair. *'Twixt Sirdar and Menelik: An Account of a Year's Expedition from Zeila to Cairo Through Unknown Abyssinia*. New York: Negro Universities Press, 1969.

Wilson, Peter J. "Status Ambiguity and Spirit Possession." *Man* 2, (1967): 366–78.

Wood, John. *When Men Are Women: Manhood Among Gabra Nomads of East Africa*. Madison: The University of Wisconsin Press, 1999.

World Population Prospects: The 1996 Revision. United Nations, 1997.

Zegeye, Abebe, and Siegfried Pausewang. *Ethiopia in Change: Peasantry, Nationalism and Democracy*. London; New York: British Academic Press; In the U.S.A. and Canada distributed by St. Martin's Press, 1994.

Zekaria, Ahmed. "Hyena Porridge: Ethnographic Filming in the City of Harar." *Sociology Ethnology Bulletin* 1 No. 1 (1992): 86–93.

———. "Harari Basketry through the Eyes of Amina Ismael Sherif." In *Ethiopia: Traditions of Creativity*, edited by Raymond Silverman, 47–64. Seattle: University of Washington Press, 1999.

———. Personal Communication. October 12, 1999.

———. "Some Notes on the Account-Book of Amir 'Abd Al-Shakur B. Yusuf (1783–1794) of Harar." *Sudanic Africa* 8 (1997): 17–36.

Zewde, Bahru. *The Ethiopian Intelligentsia and the Italo–Ethiopian War 1935–1941.* Discussion Papers in the African Humanities, Boston: African Studies Center Boston University, 1991.

———. *A History of Modern Ethiopia 1855–1974.* London: James Curry Ltd, 1991.

Interviews (oral sources)
(All names are abbreviated to protect anonymity)

A.A.J. (F). Alla Oromo. Age: 80. April 4, 2000; May 16, 17, 2010. Harar, Ethiopia.

A.G.M. (F). Kutayyee Argobba. Age: 30. March 5, 2000; May 16, 2010. Harar, Ethiopia.

A.H.T. (M). Hawwiyya Somali. Age: 77. March 18, 2000. Baabile, Ethiopia.

A.I. (M). Nole Oromo. Age: 62. February 14, 2000. Baabile, Ethiopia.

A.K. (F). Alla Oromo. Age: 65. March 27, 2000; June 15, 2003. Harar, Ethiopia.

A.M. (M). Alla Oromo. Age: 45. April 6, 2000. Harar, Ethiopia.

A.S. (M). Harari. Age: unknown. February 10, 2000; May 20, 2010. Harar, Ethiopia.

A.S.J. (M). Alla Oromo. Age: 31. July 1998. Addis Ababa, Ethiopia. October 6, 10, 11, 29, 1999. Addis Ababa, Ethiopia. February 9, 16, 28, 2000. Harar, Ethiopia.

A.S.I. (F). Arsi Oromo. Age: 45. February 25, 2000; March 11, 2000; May 5, 2010. Awwaday, Ethiopia.

A.Y. (M). Nole Oromo. Age: 50. February 20, 2000. Dire Dawa, Ethiopia.

B.F.I. (M). Girii Somali. Age: 50. March 18, 2000. Baabile, Ethiopia.

B.K. (M). Alla Oromo. Age: 32. October 10, 1999; November 16, 2000; June 7, 12, 2000. Addis Ababa, Ethiopia.

B.M.A. (F). Kutayyee Argobba. Age: 35. March 5, 2000. Harar, Ethiopia.

C.F. (F). Amhara. Age: late 20s. February 15, 2000. Baabile, Ethiopia.

D.A. (F). Anniya Oromo. Age: 17. March 7, 28, 2000; April 10, 2000. AwWoday, Ethiopia.

F.A.Q. (F). Kutayyee Argobba. Age: 30. March 5, 2000. Harar, Ethiopia.

G.F. (F). Arsi Oromo. Age: 35. April 17, 2010. Shashemene, Ethiopia.

H.S.O. (M). Wallo Oromo. Age: 55. May 9, 2010. Kemise, Ethiopia.

I.A. (M). Nole Oromo. Age: 52. February 20, 2000; June 16, 2003; May 6, 2010. Dire Dawa, Ethiopia.

I.M. (F). Arsi Oromo. Age: 17. March 7, 27, 28, 2000; April 10, 2000; November 10, 2001. AwWoday, Ethiopia; May 28, 29, 2010 East Leigh, Kenya.

J.A. (M). Jarso Oromo. Age: 65. February 3, 2000. Jarso, Ethiopia.

K.A.M. (F). Ala Oromo. Age: 50. March 12, 2000, April 12, 14, 2000. Harar, Ethiopia.

K.U. (F). Nole Oromo. Age: 36. February 14, 28, 2000. Baabile, Ethiopia.

M.A. (F). Jarso Oromo. Age: 65. February 3, 2000. Jarso, Ethiopia.